AF682236

A THERAPIST'S HANDBOOK TO DISSOLVE SHAME AND DEFENSE

Master the Moment

The effort to surmount shame and formidable defenses in psychotherapy can trigger shame and self-doubt in therapists. Susan Warren Warshow offers a user-friendly-guide to help therapists move past common treatment barriers. This unique book avoids jargon and breaks down complex concepts into digestible elements for practical application. The core principles of Dynamic Emotional Focused Therapy (DEFT), a comprehensive treatment approach for demonstrable change, are illustrated with rich and abundant clinical vignettes.

This engaging, often lyrical handbook emphasizes "shame-sensitivity" to create the safety necessary to achieve profound interpersonal connection. Often overlooked in treatment, shame can undermine the entire process. The author explains the "therapeutic transfer of compassion for self," a relational phenomenon that purposefully generates affective expression. She introduces a three-step, robust framework, the Healing Triad, to orient therapists to intervene effectively when the winds of resistance arise. Chapters clarify:

- Why we focus on feelings
- How to identify and move beyond shame and anxiety
- Transforming toxic guilt into reparative actions
- Disarming defenses while avoiding ruptures.

This book is essential reading for both advanced and newly practicing mental health practitioners striving to access the profound emotions in their clients for transformative change.

Susan Warren Warshow, LCSW (Licensed Clinical Social Worker), LMFT (Licensed Marriage & Family Therapist), is the founder of the Dynamic Emotion Focused Therapy Institute (DEFT), an international presenter, a faculty member of the ISTDP Institute (Intensive Short-Term Dynamic Psychotherapy), and a Certified IEDTA Teacher/Supervisor (International Experiential Dynamic Therapy Association). She has published several professional journal articles. She treats individuals and couples and offers clinical supervision.

She has presented at the Brief Therapy Conferences, IEDTA biennial international conferences, SEPI (Society for the Exploration of Psychotherapy Integration) and NASW (National Association of Social Workers) conferences, several Los Angeles County Psychological Association conventions and chapters of the California Association of Marriage and Family Therapists. She has lectured at California State University Northridge, California Graduate Institute, and the California School of Professional Psychology.

Her former employment includes Psychotherapist, Supervisor and Coordinator of Continuing Education at the Department of Psychiatry at Northridge Hospital. At the Center for the Improvement of Child Caring, she produced over 100 public presentations on child abuse and neglect in L.A. County and was the media director for L.A.'s first child abuse hotline.

"The Dynamic Emotion Focused therapy of Susan Warshow spotlights advances in psychotherapy that bring new luster to the clinical work of both doyens and tyros. Clear, concise writing and illuminating transcripts sharpen the realization of practical principles. The author is an expert who will enliven the development of your expertise."

Jeffrey K. Zeig, *PhD, The Milton H. Erickson Foundation*

"Doing psychotherapy is a paradox. All day, every day, you are with people. And yet, when it comes to helping your client in the moment, you are utterly alone. *A Therapist's Handbook to Dissolve Shame and Defense* fills the void. Like a wise mentor, Susan Warren Warshow senses the challenges you will face and steps in with sage advice."

Scott D. Miller, *PhD, Director, International Center for Clinical Excellence*

"If you are a therapist struggling personally and professionally in client sessions, read Susan Warren Warshow. She offers a practical guide with ample vignettes for clinicians who feel stuck yet have the courage to slow down and start making subtle, significant shifts to strengthen their skills."

Dr. Stan Tatkin, *PsyD, MFT, author of Wired for Love and We Do*

"Every therapist faces the challenge of how to empathize with the wholeness of the patient: her longings, anxiety, and the behaviors that prevent her from fulfilling her deepest desires. In *A Therapist's Handbook to Dissolve Shame and Defense*, Susan Warshow beautifully illustrates through numerous vignettes how to help patients face avoided feelings and move beyond anxiety and defenses that prevent them from pursuing their passions. For any therapist who wants to deepen their capacity for empathy, compassion, and deeper healing, this book is a must read."

Jon Frederickson, *MSW, Faculty, Washington School of Psychiatry; Author of Co-Creating Change, The Lies We Tell Ourselves, and Co-Creating Safety: Healing the Fragile Client*

"With wisdom and clarity, Susan Warshow provides key concepts to enable clinicians to work effectively with shame—both our own and that of our patients. Referring to shame as 'the gatekeeper in therapy', she provides moving clinical vignettes to illustrate its powerful role in development, its relationship to anxiety, its protective signal function for survival. Rather than attacking shame, she teaches us how to guide patients in recognizing shame and to make use of the transformative power of compassion."

Pamela J. McCrory, *PhD, Licensed Psychologist PSY 12094; Assistant Clinical Professor, Department of Psychiatry and Biobehavioral Sciences, UCLA David Geffen School of Medicine; Co-Chair, Arts, Creativity and Culture Committee, Los Angeles County Psychological Association*

"Susan Warshow's book offers an essential contribution to psychotherapists and students in clinical settings, focusing on the centrality of shame in emotional suffering. She highlights psychotherapy elements that facilitate greater self-acceptance and social intimacy. Well-chosen client examples bring her conceptualizations to life and demonstrate the nuances of an attuned approach to working with shame and defense in psychotherapy.

Her honest personal sharing accents the book in a thought-provoking way, and her astute insights are free of unnecessary jargon. *A Therapist's Handbook to Dissolve Shame and Defense* amplifies that shame is a gateway to emotional integration. Many authors theorize about the meaning of compassion. However, this book demonstrates what this profoundly important phenomenon looks like in actual therapeutic encounters. *A Therapist's Handbook to Dissolve Shame and Defense* speaks more to being present, gently challenging, and leaning into the shame experiences that emerge not only in the client but also in the therapist. How the therapist meets that difficult emotion is key, and the overall premise is that one cannot be present to the shame in another if one cannot face those experiences within oneself. Her gift to therapists is to encourage authenticity, and she has generously offered her own processes as the conduit for showing the way."

Juliet Rohde-Brown, *PhD; Chair, Depth Psychology: Integrative Therapy and Healing Practices Specialization, Pacifica Graduate Institute; Licensed Clinical Psychologist*

"Susan Warren Warshow's book is a must read for every clinician! The author's compassion shines through every page. Elegantly written in simple language, her personal style sinks under theory to reveal embodied exchanges within the nitty gritty of emotional healing. Warshow offers the wisdom and humility of a seasoned practitioner alongside the courage to reveal insecurities and vulnerabilities that inevitably emerge when working with the deepest wounds to the self."

Terry Marks-Tarlow, *PhD; Private practice in Santa Monica, California; Conducts workshops and trainings internationally; Author of A Fractal Epistemology for a Scientific*

Psychology (2020, Cambridge Scholars), *Play & Creativity in Psychotherapy* (2017), *Awakening Clinical Intuition* (2014, Norton), and *Clinical Intuition in Psychotherapy* (2012, Norton)

"Susan Warren Warshow has written a valuable book to guide therapists deeper into the life-changing alliance with their clients that fosters enthusiasm and real growth for both participants. Covering all the important bases of resistance, anxiety, guilt, shame, and especially compassion, Warshow offers detailed process descriptions of her Dynamic Emotion Focused Therapy (DEFT), providing succinct in-session transcripts of meaningful therapeutic exchanges and outcomes. *A Therapist's Handbook to Dissolve Shame and Defense* is an inspiring book to read, to reflect on, and to savor the warmth and wisdom emanating from each page."

Stella Resnick, *PhD; Author of Body-to-Body Intimacy: Transformation through Love, Sex, and Neurobiology (2019); Creator of the Embodied Relational Sex Therapy (ERST) training*

"*A Therapist's Handbook to Dissolve Shame and Defence: Master the Moment* is clinical brilliance at its best. Essential components of excellent therapeutic communication skills are expertly described here, and unpacked with useful true-to-life clinical examples. Therapeutic exchanges highlight the use of effective thought empathy and feeling empathy, so essential for the therapeutic process, especially when interfacing with those who are exploring deeply hidden aspects of shame and remorse.

Warshow demonstrates how she shares her own feelings in a caring, honest, supportive, and fruitful way. Her many metaphorical examples underscore how the therapist can effectively nudge the client in assisting the change process while at the same time honouring and respecting the importance of gently and patiently moving forward at the client's pace.

A treasury of heartfelt approaches and interventions that transcend all theoretical schools of thought, this book is one that can be read over and over by both novice and seasoned professional alike, each time finding more value, and adding to one's ability to effectively master the clinical moment with skill, kindness, and warmth."

Karin S. Hart, *PsyD; Licensed Psychologist; Former Assistant Clinical Professor, Department of Psychiatry and Biobehavioral Sciences, UCLA David Geffen School of Medicine*

A THERAPIST'S HANDBOOK TO DISSOLVE SHAME AND DEFENSE

Master the Moment

Susan Warren Warshow

Routledge
Taylor & Francis Group
NEW YORK AND LONDON

First published 2022
by Routledge
605 Third Avenue, New York, NY 10158

and by Routledge
2 Park Square, Milton Park, Abingdon, Oxon, OX14 4RN

Routledge is an imprint of the Taylor & Francis Group, an informa business

© 2022 Taylor & Francis

The right of Susan Warren Warshow to be identified as author of this work has been asserted by her in accordance with sections 77 and 78 of the Copyright, Designs and Patents Act 1988.

All rights reserved. No part of this book may be reprinted or reproduced or utilized in any form or by any electronic, mechanical, or other means, now known or hereafter invented, including photocopying and recording, or in any information storage or retrieval system, without permission in writing from the publishers.

Trademark notice: Product or corporate names may be trademarks or registered trademarks, and are used only for identification and explanation without intent to infringe.

Library of Congress Cataloging-in-Publication Data
A catalog record for this title has been requested

ISBN: 9780367024383 (hbk)
ISBN: 9780367024390 (pbk)
ISBN: 9780429399633 (ebk)

DOI: 10.4324/9780429399633

Typeset in Joanna
by KnowledgeWorks Global Ltd.

Helen and Hausie
Precious Parents
You taught me to believe in myself

Darling Donn
Beloved Husband, Wise Friend
Your wit and love lift my spirits daily

CONTENTS

FOREWORD

A Therapist's Handbook to Dissolve Shame and Defense: Master the Moment brings a unique and innovative voice to the field of psychotherapy, offering therapists a richly conceptualized, comprehensive approach to the formidable obstacles we face daily. Susan painstakingly elaborates the features of *shame sensitive* therapy, deepening relational safety to support the risk-taking necessary for change to occur in treatment. She also assists therapists to move into an internal state of compassion, a key element of her transformative work.

When I hear from a new patient that they've been in treatment for years without satisfactory results, my hope for a positive outcome intensifies. Susan provides a clear and practical guide for clinicians with profoundly touching session vignettes to illustrate how she engages her clients to move beneath their defenses, shame, anxiety, and guilt to reach new and fulfilling emotional connection and healing.

As healers, we must face the wounded aspects of ourselves that trigger fears of failure and rejection, avoidance of emotional intimacy, pressures to perform and succeed. We must use the same skill-set our clients receive and find the courage to do our inner work. Susan conveys an exceptional tenderness toward her fellow clinicians, with particular sensitivity to our vulnerable and challenging journey. She wrote this book for us, hoping to generate self-compassion as we face universal fears and doubts. She recognizes that when we are blocked, we are less able to help others and emphasizes the therapist's healing as much as the client's.

In addition to looking at our struggles and limitations, therapists must also be willing to question our clinical skills, even our favorites, when we hit rough patches or outcomes are less than envisioned. With this in mind, I've been a lifelong learner, eager to incorporate whatever works. Because there's no such thing as one size fits all, I ask myself, "What am I missing? What could I do better?" I ask my patients "What did you find useful today?" "What was not helpful?" I believe that all clinicians do better by listening, learning, and experimenting.

Susan is an artist of psychotherapy integration. Her approach, Dynamic Emotion Focused Therapy, brings together psychodynamic theory, intersubjective theory, attachment-based theory, and moment-to-moment somatic tracking. Key to her work is an emphasis on authenticity, collaborative engagement, clinical intuition, and embodied attunement to create the highest quality relationships possible.

A Therapist's Handbook to Dissolve Shame and Defense: Master the Moment is an exquisitely sensitive and effective guide to emotionally focused work. Session transcripts will take you straight to the heart of the matter as you watch a gentle but tenacious therapist help her clients face the unfaceable. Chapter by chapter will introduce you to user-friendly principles and skills that foster a robust working alliance and clear the path to emotional freedom.

Susan Warshow's book is beautifully written with a perfect dose of humility and self-revelation, a gift to the therapy literature.

Diana Shulman, PhD
Author, *ABCs of Love: Learn How Couples Rekindle Desire and Get Happy Again*

ACKNOWLEDGMENTS

My mother, Helen, taught me that people wanted acknowledgment more than anything. She emphasized listening attentively to make all people feel important. Her wisdom is a driving force in my life. My heart breaks that she cannot be here to share this book's publication. Her joy would have been immense. My dad, Hausie, showed me that my dreams were possible. My sister, Linda, always stands by me.

My darling husband, Donn Warshow, PhD, is my soulmate and best friend. He embodies joy and playfulness, bringing a rich dimensionality to our relationship. His steadfast support is rock solid, and his input on the book has been invaluable. We share our professional journeys, and he keeps me regulated through the strongest winds. This book could not exist without him.

How do I acknowledge my right hand, Bridget Quebodeaux, LMFT? Bridget is the DEFT Institute Training Director, and her presence is on every page. Her meticulous research assistance and attention to detail enrich this book. She taught me how therapists could best absorb my teachings and nudges me to present my ideas in digestible ways. She loves lists, so I created many of them! Her infinite giving astounds me. We share a love for this work and each other.

Jon Frederickson has been my treasured mentor for two decades. His faith in me gave me the confidence to teach and write. I am in awe of his dedication to this book. As busy as he is, he worked tirelessly to help me edit. Although I would cringe at his delete notations, they substantially improved the quality of the writing. Jon is a prolific author. Peers have described his books as "masterworks" that are "destined to be classics." He is a consummate clinician and international trainer.

My distinguished ISTDP trainers (Robert Neborsky, MD, Patricia Coughlin Della-Selva, PhD, Allan Abbass, MD, and Josette ten Have-de Labije, PsyD.) changed the course of my career, and I will always be grateful for their brilliant contributions to my understanding of the change forces in psychotherapy.

This book stands on the shoulders of my dear friends and colleagues who have believed in me. Diana Shulman, PhD, refueled my spirits during times of doubt and discouragement. Terry Marks-Tarlow, PhD, shared her immense insight and writing experience. Ron Fouts, my professional coach, lovingly nurtured this book. I profoundly appreciate the unwavering support of Juliet Rhode-Brown, PhD, Pamela McCrory, PhD, Karin Hart, PhD, Scott Miller, PhD, Stella Resnick, PhD, Barbara Wilson, LCSW, Bruce Ammons, PhD, Sherry Cook, and Sharrell Blakeley, MSW. They hold a special place in my heart. Dr. Allan Schore immensely enriched my understanding of neuroscience and validated my clinical instincts as a participant in his study group.

My clients and trainees have brought a richness to my life I could not have imagined. I cherish each one. They have inspired me to stretch my boundaries and taught me to love in infinite new ways. I thank God for the privilege of working in this profession and providing daily inspiration in my practice, teaching, and writing.

INTRODUCTION

Sitting on Therapeutic Gold

The idea for this book sprung into my mind after I'd given two Saturday workshops for therapists in LA and Pasadena. I didn't expect the many enthusiastic comments about the comprehensive handouts I'd created for the attendees. Two ongoing training groups formed from those events, and I decided to use the handouts for our source material. My trainees never showed up without their booklets in hand, and their copies were dog-eared and scribbled throughout with copious notes. I was amazed at comments like, "I keep this with me all the time to read right before my sessions," and "I study the part that applies to a particular client the day before the appointment." I thought, "Why not publish this handout in its raw form and make it available to other therapists too?" But I don't make anything easy. Over the years, the handout morphed into the book you're reading, written for psychotherapists who work daily on the front lines of psychological trauma. My trainees have asked me to write a book for years. They presented me with a touching album entitled *For Your Journey*, with photos, quotes, and personal comments to encourage my writing. The album opens with, "Susan, as you continue to walk with us, so we wish to walk with you—as you write your life's work, as you share the fruits of your labor, as you do all that matters to your heart. Take our words, take our wishes, take our love with you always on all your journeys." My trainees inspired me to pass on the fertile and practical wisdom I've gathered over the years. I dedicate this book to them and all therapists who dream of bringing a better life to others.

DOI: 10.4324/9780429399633-1

If you had told me I would one day teach therapists and write a book for them, you could have said I'd become an astronaut. For most of my professional career, I did not see beyond my private practice. Let me take you back to a day in my office many years ago. My client had asked, "How can you sit and listen to people's problems all day?" It was hard enough for him to talk about his emotional suffering for an hour a week, much less imagine how I could sit with people's anguish every day. When the session ended, he pulled up from his chair, waved goodbye, and headed to Los Angeles International Airport to catch a flight to Milan. He was a businessman with interests around the world. As the door closed behind him, I looked around my four walls and felt envious. His life looked far more colorful than mine, although surface comparisons were illusory. His inner world was chaotic. Nevertheless, his last question triggered my teenage fantasy of becoming a photojournalist.

Why did I choose this work? Perhaps because I sensed something wordlessly beautiful about the privilege to create a life-changing connection with another human being? However, once I got into the nitty-gritty of daily practice, "life-changing" didn't always happen. Like my trainees today, I craved specific guidance when I faced confounding setbacks, such as when a client's explosive outbursts, which had been under control, returned with a vengeance and put his marriage on the brink. Or someone who had stabilized dove suddenly into depressive hell. My body would retract and retreat into my overstuffed chair. As the therapeutic "flow" reversed direction, I'd watch hard work evaporate through the air vents, and the arduous process would begin anew.

Treatment roadblocks are especially problematic with clients who have complicated histories of multiple traumas and entrenched self-sabotaging patterns. Many clients told me they had tried other therapies with disappointing results. This profile fits a lot of people who seek our help! These clients appeared to need more than new cognitive habits, empathic responding, analytical insight, pure catharsis, temporary relief from anxiety, or trauma incident resolution to produce a fundamental, lasting shift within themselves. One small issue remained. For years, I didn't know what an alternative approach would be!

When I felt stuck, I'd dig around my tool bag, like one of my overstuffed handbags, searching for that piece of information that would move the process forward. If I came up empty, I'd once again feel frustrated with the ambiguity of psychotherapy. After so many years of training, how could I still be unclear? Which of the often-conflicting theories should I rely upon in the face of the immediate challenge? Why do some approaches work with certain clients but not others, and how many methods do I need to learn? Will it ever be good enough? I was impatient with therapies that achieved limited goals or required interminably long periods of time. I hoped my clients didn't notice my shame and anxiety as we both sat with the uncertainty I'd come to expect. Rationales like, "It takes a person many years to become who they are, and it will take years for change to occur," did not make the process more palatable.

Sometimes we think we know what's going on with the client, but when we're misattuned, we see a higher dropout rate. A large-scale, 15-year study of psychotherapists showed that almost half lacked confidence in their therapeutic strategies, their ability to gain their client's cooperation in the therapeutic task, and doubted their understanding of what was happening moment by moment during their sessions (Orlinsky & Ronnestad, 2005). Another study (550 cases) indicated that lab tests and algorithms predicted client deterioration more effectively than 48 therapists (Hannan et al., 2005). I lacked confidence more than I would have liked, and it was comforting to know I wasn't the only one.

My excitement for my work slipped over the years. I mused about people who had jobs like carpentry or hairstyling, as they could see results quickly. A carpenter didn't have to wonder if he'd finished a cabinet. In contrast, the stack of continuing education brochures that papered my bulletin board collectively howled, "You don't know enough, and you never will!" I tried to wrap my brain around the idea of being a "good enough" therapist, but I wanted more, which caused me to seek continuing education beyond the amount required for my license. But brilliant lectures often become abstractions when I sat across from a challenging client.

A Radical Shift

A new development in our field threatened to upend my practice as I had known it. The insurance industry exerted pressure to make psychotherapy more cost-effective.

From the New York Times:

> Many therapists say managed-care companies, intent on cutting costs, are undermining the quality of care by calling the shots on treatment without ever seeing a patient. These companies, they say, favor doctors who charge the lowest fees, driving some practitioners from the profession.
>
> "This industry is destroying the field," said Karen Shore, psychologist, and co-chairwoman of the Coalition of Mental Health Professionals and Consumers. This Long Island-based national group opposes managed care for mental health. "Nobody wants their kid to be a psychologist anymore."
>
> (Henneberger, 1994, p. 1)

An officious, not-so-gentle man from one of the managed care companies spoke at a luncheon meeting, and he told our group of quaking therapists that "we would no longer determine the course of client treatment." He also said that approximately 80% of us would be unemployed in private practice within five years. This impending threat spawned a deluge of workshops, and my survival instincts heightened my interest in "Brief Therapy." A conference caught my eye at the University of California at Los Angeles (UCLA), led by a Harvard educated psychiatrist and psychoanalyst from Montreal, Dr. Habib Davanloo, the father of Intensive Short-Term Dynamic Psychotherapy (ISTDP). I might find an answer in a depth therapy that also promised to be short-term. That should do the trick!

To my amazement, Dr. Davanloo presented full-session videos. I was accustomed to presenters reading papers. While I learned from these lectures, I found that process notes did not advance my practical skills as well as watching session recordings. I learned more with all-senses-on-board. As I watched Davanloo's work, it felt like a strong wind was blowing me backward, or perhaps forward. Davanloo had studied thousands of his recorded sessions, asking his patients for feedback about what worked and what had not. He facilitated changes I would not have believed possible in initial three-hour trial therapies. How does a client who has lived his life in a shut-down mode allow himself to release rage and break into sobs in the first session? I was amazed at the work, yet I also found it anxiety producing and unfamiliar. I told my husband, "This work is incredible, but I'll never practice this approach." Curiosity took me to subsequent conferences. Five years later, I would train in ISTDP (Davanloo, 2001), which richly informs my work.

While I felt enormously excited about my new skills, I also experienced more ruptures in my practice, as resistance to emotional closeness pushed back my efforts to reach affect. I became aware that shame was the primary barrier that stood in the way of more consistent positive responses. When I addressed shame as self-attack, many clients saw this as a deficiency within them. Attempts at an explanation didn't seem to help. I had to find ways to transcend shame.

I developed a Dynamic Emotion Focused Therapy (DEFT) model that puts *shame sensitivity* work (Chapter 6), the Healing Triad: Bypassing Treatment Barriers (Chapter 5), and the Therapeutic Transfer of Compassion for Self (Chapter 5) at its center. I view compassion as the antidote to shame. People who seek our help don't have high self-care and lack awareness of unconscious forces that disable them. The therapist offers a rare type of caring, embracing the person before us and the individual who is yet to emerge. I chose the DEFT acronym to emphasize the emotion focused and psychodynamic foundations of this approach. I also liked the deft synonyms: adroit, expert, skillful, proficient, nimble, masterly, and artful.

I could not have foreseen the conversion of forces that would reignite my early passion again. When clients recognize the internal operations that disable them, absorb the therapist's compassion, and experience a partnership that makes alternatives possible, change begins. However, both the client and the therapist must nurture compassion within themselves for this process to take place. Metaphorically, we couldn't offer brownies until we'd baked them, and others couldn't enjoy the brownies until they ingested them. The therapist must "bake" her compassion before she can offer it.

The following is a transcript of a supervisory session. The therapist describes to me her internal process to awaken compassion within herself while working with a young mother:

Th: My client devalues her child relentlessly. I felt myself pulling back from her and not liking her. Suddenly, I was able to change how I felt. I said to myself, 'Oh, my goodness. I see what is meant by the 'Therapeutic Transfer of Compassion for Self!' There was this moment where I pulled my attention toward my client as a little kid, remembering all the things that I know had happened to her. I recalled the way her father treated her with contempt, and

> I just had this real experience of a connection to her. I teared up, and I stopped judging her. I felt true compassion for her, and she completely shifted. She not only shifted the way she was talking about herself, but she said, 'Oh! I'm doing to my daughter what my father did to me.' And I hadn't said anything! She just shifted the minute I shifted. It was pretty amazing."

When I raised a couple's awareness of the harm caused by the husband's intellectualization and the wife's withdrawal, they were stunned. When they became able to see how these defenses led to their separation and that they could let go of them, they both expressed significant relief and hope. Although both partners were easily wounded and ready to flee, they could look at their defenses without becoming more defensive because I was sensitive to their shame. The wife wanted more closeness, and the husband didn't think he could feel. When I told him that he could name an emotion with one word, and his (excessive) verbalizations got in his way, he saw the difference between a thought and a feeling with clarity. He was flabbergasted. He said no one ever made that distinction in years of therapy, meaning that no one had helped him become aware of his intellectualizing defense or its alternative. His body turned 180 degrees toward her, and he expressed his fear without a deluge of words. She lifted her wall and cried. At that moment, a new relationship began.

My developing framework caused most clients to exclaim that they'd never felt so understood. I was deeply touched when fragile and determinedly defended clients revealed themselves as never before. Richard, a tightly restrained young man with piercing eyes, allowed tears to stream down his cheeks in the course of our first session. He'd thanked me because he'd come to believe that he couldn't feel anything.

I began identifying core principles that held up well under the pressure of day to day practice. The client's own words provided the most valuable assessment of the process. I credit Dr. Davanloo and Dr. Scott Miller for making me mindful of seeking client feedback in every session. They inspired me to make it a point to frequently inquire after or during sessions, "Please share with me how this session (or exchange) has been for you?" "Please tell me what worked and anything that didn't." "What might you use from today?" Throughout the session, I'd ask, "How does my comment land with you?" "Please tell me how you understand what I've said" or "Do you feel I've understood what you've said?" My inquiries allowed me to do my own informal research, and I gathered considerable information from my clients that I put to good use.

I felt compelled to share what I was learning with my colleagues. One client, a beloved teacher and a psychologist, told me that she "wanted out" of her profession. The idea of retirement brought her a feeling of liberation. But why? She didn't want the "intensity" anymore. She agonized over treatment failures and gave little credit to the ways she'd impacted others. Exploration showed that her self-judgments catapulted her into agitated states during those times when she couldn't help those clients who put faith in her. Unresolved struggles in her practice drove her to want to exit. I write this book for her and others who feel like her, as I once did.

Perhaps she would have felt less discouraged had she discovered the accelerated emotional intimacy and clearer orientation to conflict resolution that I found to be possible. Mason, a charismatic, gifted, and depressed man with a trail of relationship wreckage behind him, held contempt for dependency needs and was proud of his warrior mentality. Inspiring him to change course was like turning a freighter in the opposite direction in a narrow canal. Amazingly, he finally took the risk of exposing his fears and unmet yearnings to me, sometimes sobbing or releasing rage. Eventually, he started bravely exposing his vulnerable feelings to significant others. I opened my email recently to find this message from him, "I woke up this morning with a beautiful feeling of relationship with others." My heart sang.

In my programs and presentations, I show session recordings in which I work with a spectrum of psychoneurosis to therapists worldwide who practice diverse psychotherapy models. Many tell me they love their models while also seeing something in my work that is new and desirable for them. The profound emotional connections emerging in the early sessions move them. They sometimes express shame. When one seasoned therapist said to me, "I need to up my game," she had pain on her face. I have felt the same many times. Psychologists, psychiatrists, psychotherapists, and interns have shared poignant stories about their professional and personal difficulties practicing therapy. I feel great affection and appreciation for their sincere devotion, touching vulnerabilities, and bravery.

My fellow clinicians who have attended my programs shaped this book. They've shown me where they're stuck and how I can help them.

Trainees push me to provide practical, clear, and immediately applicable interventions. Consequently, I've developed numerous skill-building role-plays. I've groaned many times when asked to do more to make further clarifications, but I try to remember that life is always a journey.

As I sat with a client one day, I had the exact thought, "I'm sitting on therapeutic gold!" I wrote a blog soon after with that title. The foundational principles I discuss in this book created a seismic change in my work and gave me new clarity when dealing with treatment barriers. Two clients with severe avoidant patterns come to mind. Both were single and isolated into their 50's, and they yearned for relationships. The work with them was gradual, but one is now married, and the other has an abundance of friends who adore her. Both described themselves as happy. I don't believe I could have facilitated these characterological changes without the therapeutic approach I'm about to share.

This "Handbook" offers immediate, practical guidance to the clinician. I want to be real and avoid overinflating expectations. Lifelong defenses don't disappear entirely, and in times of acute stress, regressions occur in anyone's life. But when the client is willing to go to work with the therapist, there is cause for real optimism. Session vignettes will illustrate how shifts in attachment, trust, and intimacy patterns can evolve in an accelerated manner. While long term work is beneficial for many, I hope to illuminate how we can plant seeds of change moment to moment, a new kernel with a life of its own.

Relief as the Mist Lifts

Our therapeutic orientations organize how we will react to chaotic, rapidly emerging phenomena in session. When we clearly "see" and respond accurately to the obstacles to connection in the moment, we do our part to promote progress. Either therapy partner can feel overwhelmed by the complexity of phenomena arising in a session, and this book offers practical guidance to meet a broad range of challenges. Practicing this work necessitates that we slow down to sharpen our focus and our senses. Moment-to-moment tracking is like using a telephoto lens. Everything recedes except the image in the forefront. Multiple layers of awareness still operate, but at the moment, we immerse ourselves in the Now. A therapist told me my work seems simple and organic. The key is taking one step at a time. I might say to a client, "Hold on, please. I don't want to miss what you just said." One hyper-aroused client told me he hated my slowness. He'd been in therapy since he was a kid and was impatient. Years later, he told me I was the best therapist he'd had. When we insist on not rushing, we begin to see a detail, a veiled meaning, a clue to something prescient that would have escaped our notice otherwise.

A young man who helped me edit session videos observed two of my clients during the first session and at termination, and he asked me innocently, "These aren't the same people, right?" I answered, "Yes." He shook his head vigorously, saying, "No way!" Their posture, facial coloring, and other changes in physical appearance and confidence made them unrecognizable to him. I felt compelled to share the path that led to such progress with my fellow clinicians. To not do so seemed selfish. This book is for you.

References

Davanloo, H. (2001). *Intensive short-term dynamic psychotherapy: Selected papers of Habib Davanloo.* Wiley.

Merriam-Webster. (n.d.). Deft. In *Merriam-Webster.com dictionary.* Retrieved September 1, 2010, from https://www.merriam-webster.com/dictionary/deft

Hannan, C., Lambert, M., Harmon, C., Neilsen, S., Smart, D., Schimokawa, K., & Sutton, S. (2005). A lab test and algorithms for identifying cases at risk for treatment failure. *Journal of Clinical Psychology, 61*(2), 155–163. https://doi.org/10.1002/jclp.20108

Henneberger, M. (1994, October 9). Managed care changing practice of psychotherapy. *The New York Times.* http://www.nytimes.com

Orlinsky, D. E., & Ronnestad, M. H. (2005). *How psychotherapists develop: A study of therapeutic work and professional growth.* American Psychological Association.

1

THE WARRIOR THERAPIST

The warrior therapist that I envision does not overpower, bully, push, or show aggression in any way. Warrior therapists risk fear and loss for the sake of love. They must reach for reserves of strength and courage within themselves to help their clients battle the forces that destroy their lives. I found that I needed bravery to grapple with my own internal barriers in this process. "I believe great power exists in the warrior stance as it translates clinically to the embrace of uncertainty. During. psychotherapy, this means not having to know that which cannot yet be known. To adopt this mental attitude allows us to remain emotionally open, cognitively poised and spiritually strong enough to withstand the heat of intense emotion, confusion, even delusion in our patients, not to mention ourselves." (Tarlow, T.M., 2012) When I began practicing with intensely emotion focused therapy, I feared the feelings that might be encountered and mishandled in a session. What if I were to alienate my client? Although people want change, habitual patterns of self-protection prefer to remain entrenched. Working with resistance requires risk-taking and tolerance for uncertainty. Racker writes, "The neurotic is a prisoner of his resistances and needs constant and intense help from the [therapist] if he is to liberate himself from his chains" (Racker, 1968, p. 178). The warrior

DOI: 10.4324/9780429399633-2

therapist must take chances to support the client's will to be free from shaming, punitive, and restrictive barriers. Resistances can lead to attacks on the therapist as well as the client. In my learning process, I had to face my fears so my clients could face theirs. The self-protective system, designed to ward off rejection and injury in the past, would rebuff my attempts to help in the present.

With permission from my client, I would reflect reality even when painful, trusting and sharing my perceptions in a more real, sensitive and vulnerable way. I would immerse myself in my client's experiences, involving mind, body, spirit, imagery, impulses, and imagination. With a shared willingness to risk, profound unlockings of feelings became possible within hours of knowing each other. This extraordinary experience, repeated often, laid the foundation for secure attachment relationships for numerous clients.

In the following vignette, the client began our first session describing his sense of failure that he'd been unable to connect to any emotions in his prior therapy. He suffered from high social anxiety. I started by acknowledging his willingness to be vulnerable with me in the present:

Th: It takes courage to let me know your struggles, and I appreciate that. I sense and care about your pain. (*My face reveals caring. He grimaces and shakes his head with skepticism.*)

Ct: I guess I don't understand the value in that (*fidgeting with his hands*). I told Carol (*his former therapist*) very early on, I have such trouble accepting statements like that. What does that mean to me? It doesn't make me feel any better to know that you're there with me. I don't get any relief from that. I don't get any satisfaction or joy or anything from that. So, I think it should mean something to me, and I should be able to make that connection, but I don't.

Th: I'm glad you told me the truth. You don't get any satisfaction from another person caring about you?

Ct: (*He shakes his head.*) No. When I think about dating, I wonder, "Why would anybody want to be with me?"

He rebuffed my attempts to draw closer and encouraged me to feel discouraged, as he did with his ex-wife. I may be tempted to withdraw but instead chose to "take a stand for good." I face the rejecting part of him, risking more rejection, so he might see how his distancing mechanism hurts him and our relationship.

Th: Sadly, you expect rejection, Kevin, and I believe there's a viciousness toward yourself that operates within you. (*He listens attentively and nods with agreement.*) A part of you tells you that when you go online, "Why would anybody want to be with me?" It also tells you to dismiss another person's caring for you. Like mine. (*He agrees.*) And then you feel desperately alone. There's something inside you that doesn't want you to know your value or to experience your worth to others. (*He continues to fidget with hands.*)

Ct: Almost like there's another side, an evil side.

Th: A cruel side. A very cruel part that does not want you to know a caring relationship. (*He nods in agreement.*)

Ct: A cruel side. Why would that be? (*He fights back his tears.*)

Th: Yeah (*said in a whisper*). It's very sad.

Ct: (*He wipes both eyes with his left hand and keeps his eyes covered, rubbing his eyes, sighing.*) Yeah, it's sad.

Th: It's sad that you've learned to withhold caring from yourself (*he nods and bites bottom lip, eyes diverted downward in shame*), to deprive yourself, so cruelly, for many, many years.

Ct: Yeah. (*He breaks into sobs.*)

He had a full breakthrough in this three-hour session of rage, grief, guilt, and love toward a parent who taught him to hate himself. If I had backed off, as his shame and fears of closeness wanted me to do, Kevin would have lost this powerful new experience.

Another client said in an initial session, "I've had therapy before, and it never helped me. I don't believe it will now." Other dismissive comments expressing doubts about both our abilities followed. Before I became more practiced working with challenging distancing defenses, I sometimes felt overcome by them, as if this work would burn up every cell of my body. The complexity of two psyches could overwhelm me. The intersections between our lives created reverberating waves of poignant and piercing feelings, memories, and associations. The search for coherence in our two narratives seemed to extend into infinity. And then a third dimension emerged, as a newly formed relationship took shape, an entity that was neither my client nor me but us. No wonder therapists can feel lost in a labyrinth. Some avoid this vulnerable experience by claiming to be sure of their knowledge. But the path of discovery benefits from humility.

Exploring the unconscious mind is akin to illuminating the layers in the sea where light does not penetrate. "These deep zones are where we find the most bizarre and fascinating creatures in the sea. As we dive into these largely unexplored places, the temperature drops and the pressure increases at an astounding rate" (Knight, 1998). At times, the chaos of the unconscious could hit me like a massive wave, with wild sea organisms laughing at my inability to tame or make sense of them. Our shared ventures in psychotherapy take us into far-reaching layers of the fascinating and foreboding emotional memory system. Being human, both therapeutic partners have suffered varying degrees of trauma. When we get too close to unresolved pain, the shaming furies hiss and scowl and belittle us into becoming small and unseen.

In the following vignette from a second session, Brian became aware of how his mother's hatred took root in him as a young child. I help him to recognize that I see him differently than she. This session precedes profound work that scares him and would have frightened me at one time.

Ct: There's this other part I would never—I'm not going to show. I mean, I want to show. It's like dying, really. It's like dying.

Th: Hmm. Hmm. So, you hide something so vitally important inside of you, even kill it off, and reveal only the parts you feel will be safe to show me.

Ct: Well, I feel really weak. Just really weak, innocent in a way, and so fragile, really. So fragile.

Th: Hmm. What's telling you that you're weak and fragile?

Ct: I have the idea I could break down any minute. Once this thing comes up, it feels like this wave that will take everything with it. And I'm just not safe (*wiping away tears*). I'm going to drown and also it's going to be too much for others as well (*meaning me*). I'm too much for the other person. It's too much. It's like, "Go away, please." (*I counter his shame by recognizing it with compassion. He finds comfort in being seen.*)

Th: So, there's shame, a shame that you have when any of these overpowering feelings come up inside of you, as though your feelings are bad. And if they're seen by me, that I'm going to recoil, be disgusted, be overwhelmed.

Ct: Um, hum. Yeah. That's exactly right.

Th: Well, how about if we take a look? Do you see any signs of me reacting as you imagine? (*Guiding him to check out his projection of my contempt and inability to handle his feelings*).

Ct: (*Chuckling*) Okay. (*He sees reality and the absurdity of his expectation.*)

Th: What do you see?

Ct: It doesn't seem to be that way now, but I've not opened the gates.

Th: Of course. Well, why would you, when somewhere along the line, you've become convinced you're unsafe. What do you experience now with me?

Ct: You seem to be interested. My reactions don't seem to affect you negatively.

Th: Actually, I felt deep sadness when I realized how frightened you've been of your feelings since you were a young child. You link your feelings with being bad and assume you will overwhelm others who won't want you if you reveal yourself. It just felt very sad to me.

Ct: Yeah, so—

Th: Well, how does it seem to you when you look at that little boy's experience? (*It's essential that he feels caring for himself.*)

Ct: Well, on the one hand, it feels really sad to me too that he's still out there, still unacknowledged. And ashamed. And on the other hand, I want him to go away, just leave me alone.

Th: So, you see the part in you that rejects him, and it looks like it's coming from other people, like me. But Brian, something in you doesn't forgive or accept (*said with tenderness*).

Ct: Yeah. That's true. Yeah. I just, in a way, I hate that guy, you know.

His tragedy pierced me. Brian hated the child that he was. Facing the reality of his self-loathing impacted him. He agreed this had to change for our work to go forward, and he broke into sobs. To gain privileged access with a broad spectrum of people—those who shut down with shame like this man; others who push back by debating, dismissing, and belittling; and others who are consumed by anxiety—I would need bravery to speak straightforwardly about the barriers to closeness. In a short exchange, I addressed Brian's shame and his projections onto me. At an earlier time, I would not have been this clear.

For many years in my practice, I worked within my comfort zones. I made observations about my client's defensive system but failed to directly engage with it, resulting in sessions that left dysfunctional dynamics untouched. Recently a man ranted about the money he'd spent on his couple's therapy, barking that his wife hadn't changed in six months. He had anger toward our profession, which implicated our relationship. Today, I would be prepared to explore his feelings toward me, which proved to be fertile territory. Remaining in my head felt familiar and safe. I'd empathize with conscious feelings but had not discovered the path that led to the more significant unconscious emotions. I gave inadequate attention to bodily sensations and lacked a comprehensive understanding of their meaning. An example of how a therapist might skirt uncomfortable feelings occurred when I sought personal help when my mother was declining before her death. I felt overwhelmed. In the first session, I noticed butterflies in my chest and felt relief when the therapist did not draw attention to my bodily sensations. My physical discomfort embarrassed me. Yet those internal signals held the key to the necessary work that might have helped both my mother and me before she passed. Had I given voice to the fluttering in my chest, we might have uncovered my anger and desperation that she had given up on herself along with the rise of painful complex feelings.

Society and family pressure us to appear "put together," and I found it difficult to admit, "I've got some wild feelings going off in my chest." I needed my therapist's help to explore beyond the surface of my presenting problem. Could he have been intimidated too? If we don't invite the feelings behind the defenses to come forward, the client will continue to suffer. If we become passive when shame, anxiety, guilt, and self-protective strategies are activated, we unintentionally abandon the client. Yet, all therapists succumb to the defenses at times. But we can also strengthen our work by committing to the following:

The Warrior Therapist's Pledge

1 Advocate for the unspoken voices within the client
2 Reinforce the client's strengths frequently
3 Shine a light of compassion on the desire to hide and distance
4 Resist the pull to passivity when a session drifts
5 Ask probing questions with permission
6 Seek truth: reflect subjective and objective reality

7. Sustain an emotion focus once inhibitory affects are regulated
8. Face obstacles to feeling compassion for our clients
9. Overcome feeling intimidated by the defenses
10. Shift gears toward emotions as capacity increases
11. Avoid colluding with the defenses
12. Find the courage to be tenacious

Advocate for the Unspoken Voices within the Client

When our clients retreat, we actively encourage their unspoken voices. We show up as an ally, advocate, and friend to the neglected parts of the self.

> *"I noticed you started a sentence and something cut you off abruptly. Would you be willing to finish your words?"*

> *"I see the great love you have for your son and your efforts to get help for his attention-deficit/hyperactivity disorder (ADHD). In the spirit of embracing all parts of you so that your depression might lift, could we see if other feelings are there too?"*

> *"I heard something in your voice and wondered what you're feeling toward me? I think it would significantly help you to explore these feelings."*

Reinforce the Client's Strengths Frequently

Show appreciation and admiration for the client's bravery and resourcefulness. We can focus too much on what's not working and not enough on what is functional. Keep the balance in mind. Validate when the client takes risks, such as daring to disagree or challenge us. The therapist must rely on internal sources of validation and encourage the client to differentiate. This can be easier said than done.

> *"I'm glad that you told me you feel differently and disagree. I respect that we are different people."*

> *"I appreciate the courage it takes to feel the pain of your guilt for having deeply wounded your wife. I didn't realize until this moment how much you cared for her. Please allow yourself to feel your pain."*

> *"That's amazing! You asked me to stay silent while you were crying. Something you would not have done before. (I had been making soft sounds when the client held back his tears.) By telling me what you needed from me, you were able to release your grief with me. I'm so pleased you took care of yourself."*

Shine a Light of Compassion on the Desire to Hide and Distance

When a client pulls away from us, therapists may collude with the client's instincts to self-protect. But this won't help. We need to advocate for the neglected parts of the self.

> *"I have a lot of empathy as you begin to speak of this horrible experience. I also notice that you look away from me and cut off your words. May I ask if you might feel shame? I feel pain for you when something within you silences you."*

Resist the Pull to Passivity When a Session Drifts

Therapists and clients easily fall into comfortable conversations while session time runs out. Nothing shifts. Sessions come alive when a dynamic process of entering new territory is underway. Draw attention to drifting as it defeats the purpose of therapy.

> *"You are such an interesting person, and I could talk with you forever on this topic. I also care that you get what you need in our time together, and I'm wondering if we are on a path that takes you to something meaningful for you today?"*

Ask Probing Questions with Permission

Any questions that invite greater risk-taking are uncomfortable. The defensive system prefers to be undisturbed, yet our clients come to us for something new. Both therapists and clients easily settle into the status quo. Do we dare to pursue the new?

> *"You seemed to pull back from me in that moment, and you've said you want to stop withdrawing as you did with your wife. Would it be ok if we moved closer to your feelings instead of away from them and explored what you feel toward me? You have no unacceptable feelings."*

> *"I notice your hesitation when I ask how you feel about Barbara, yet your feelings are so crucial to your well-being. What is your sense of what cuts you off from yourself right now?"*

Seek Truth: Reflect Subjective and Objective Reality

Some truths are hard to acknowledge. We may take refuge in denial, minimization, and the pursuit of fantasies. But these defenses undermine the relationships we seek to build.

> *"When I mentioned I'd like to glance at my notes for a moment, you said I should have read them before the session. (The client's tone was contemptuous.) I may look at my notes, even if I've read them, to remind myself of something you said that seems very relevant now. I appreciate you telling me your perceptions, and is it ok if I do the same? (He nodded yes.)*
>
> *There was something in the way you made that comment that felt like you looked down on me. (To illustrate, I held my elbow in the air and pointed my arm downward. He nodded in agreement.) You will find flaws in me, and it's natural for you to question whether you can trust me to guide you. At the same time, I think you've come to me to help you discover parts of yourself that lie outside your awareness. If you view me as inadequate, how do you imagine this will affect your therapy?" (Said with kindness.)*

In the last example, we might be inclined to avoid conflict and begin doubting ourselves. We would lose our voice in the process, and this would erase the existence of "us." Instead, we can remember a principle: *No therapeutic work takes place when there is no relationship.* Frequently, we must find courage to discuss devaluation directly. The exchange with my client did not result in instant trust, but it did lead to a gripping session where he faced, with no further prompting from me, how he demeaned his wife. Grief broke through for the suffering he had caused her.

Sustain an Emotion Focus Once Inhibitory Affects are Regulated

Since there is always resistance to sustaining an emotion focus, therapists will need tenacity to advocate for abandoned feelings relentlessly. We will question ourselves, doubt our approach, and want to give up. Don't.

> *"May I interrupt a moment? You've said you want to be more connected to yourself. You mentioned something that happened between you and your daughter, and I can see you have strong feelings. You then brought up an acquaintance, and I wonder if we could stay with your important feelings with your daughter?"*

Face Obstacles to Feeling Compassion for Our Clients

Sometimes the greatest battle in our office is within ourselves. We want to be in a state of compassion, but we don't feel it. Therapists feel anger, disgust, and fear just like anybody else. I used to think therapists were above such reactions, and I felt surprised when a therapist sounded harsh or intolerant. That idea was naive. Of course, we're human! Facing our limitations without judgment is something we must do for ourselves before we can do it for our clients.

A therapist told me she felt anxious because she'd been angry when a client told her she was stupid, had failed her repeatedly by changing topics, and accused the therapist of manipulating her so she would spend more on sessions. The client said she was furious and knew she "had no filter." She'd verbally abused others and had driven people away. I knew this therapist was exceptionally kind and dedicated, and I felt much empathy. She was hurt and angry, and who among us can feel soft and tender at the same time? Therapists cannot sustain a state of compassion with every client at all times. This client's chronic dissatisfaction led the therapist to refer her to another clinician, whom she hoped could help her more. I helped her to see that she had the right to her feelings and to consider her well-being.

When clients are highly resistant and project frequently, it becomes vital to clarify the state of the therapeutic alliance. Here's a possible exchange when the client complained that the therapist had initiated topics that she didn't find useful:

Th: I'm noticing you were having feelings toward me as you were discussing your insomnia. I think it would help to look at what's happening with us, if you agree.

Ct: Ok. (*She says half-heartedly.*) I'm tired of talking about what goes wrong with us. I wanted to talk about my insomnia.

Th: Would you help me understand what kind of input you hope for when we discuss your insomnia? I don't want to go in any direction that you don't choose. Would you tell me your thoughts?

Ct: I've had insomnia for years. No one has been able to help. I've tried all the sleep hygiene stuff. It's a very big deal for me.

Th: I'm truly sad to hear that. Insomnia over long periods becomes agonizing. You've tried approaches that haven't helped, and you hope for something new. You've told me that your anxiety is frequently high, and you feel very disturbed at night by the instability in your relationships. I wonder if you would sleep better if your relationships felt more stable?

Ct: Probably, but people are such jerks that I don't see how that's possible.

Th: I think you're saying that if the solution to your peace of mind depends on others, then our efforts to help your insomnia are doomed. Makes sense to me. Where do we go from here? *(Addressing externalization of the problem. It's crucial to keep my comments focused on her insomnia to sustain a spirit of collaboration.)*

This client is isolated and imprisoned with no escape. That reality is tragic and evokes compassion. The therapist can offer a way out—that the client consider how she unconsciously keeps people away from her, increasing her insomnia. The same dynamic plays out in her relationship with the therapist. She successfully pushes the therapist away. They could use their relationship as an opportunity to understand how other relationships fail, perpetuating her insomnia. Or she could continue on a familiar path that leaves her alone. The choice is hers.

Overcome Feeling Intimidated by the Defenses

Self-protective strategies attempt to silence and intimidate the therapist as well as the client. Although we may be tempted, therapists never want to bully the defenses nor do we want to avoid them. The defenses become fiercer in the absence of compassion. The therapist will need to build the capacity to draw attention to the defenses with caring for the suffering they cause and allow the client to struggle with the choice to relinquish them.

Shift Gears toward Emotions as Capacity Increases

Therapists can effectively reduce dysregulated states but avoid shifting gears toward avoided feelings once anxiety drops or a defensive strategy weakens. The therapist may spend an entire session dealing with anxiety or defenses when it would be possible to move toward feelings and deeper material much sooner. We understandably become concerned about going too fast, but learning to recognize and attend to dysregulated states should give us confidence about questions of timing. I typically feel it's safe to encourage feelings when anxiety is in the striated muscles (see Figure 7.2), indicating that feelings are close to the surface and the alliance is active. When high levels of anxiety or defenses resurface, we work with those barriers until tolerance for feelings grows again.

An example of shifting gears toward emotions as a woman becomes less anxious:

"I'm so glad you're not fuzzy-headed anymore. It seems like your anxiety has dropped significantly. Do you see it that way too? *(The client agrees.)* Interesting how rapidly you became regulated with some caring attention to your anxiety. Tell me about any other sensations you notice in your body now. *(The client mentions upper arm and chest tension (striated muscle activation), which is indicative of a manageable level of anxiety.)* That's good! Your feelings are becoming more accessible. How about if we go back to your feelings toward your friend who snubbed you at the wedding?"

Bearing the fear and potential shame about the uncertainties that arise when we "shift gears" and enter the "deep zones" of feeling and imagination calls upon strengths we may not know we have. Our clients will need bravery, too, which becomes available even to the most fragile or defended person with the therapist's steady, caring presence. I often explicitly remind people that they are not alone. We can easily underestimate a client's capacity as well as our own.

Avoid Colluding with the Defenses

A distinguished, elderly professor hesitantly told me he's a cross-dresser. His lips quivered, and his eyes telegraphed fear. He had revealed his secret to only two people in his life, and he did not tell his former therapist. At this touching moment of self-disclosure, he suddenly switched to a dispassionate discussion of some articles on cross-dressing. His vulnerability had drawn me closer, but now his intellectualization created distance. His detachment had damaged several significant relationships. An opportunity presented itself to help him become aware of a silent killer of his joy. Still, the moment is sensitive. Do I interrupt him or ignore the defense? If I injure him with an insensitive comment, that would be awful. Yet I wanted to be helpful, and so I stepped up.

Th: May I interrupt for a moment? This article is informative, and I also want to share that I'm very touched by the significant risk you took in sharing your secret with me. This is a big moment! I'm wondering how it is for you to let me see you your struggles, pain, and shame about cross-dressing? I'm just feeling for you carrying this weight all these years.

Ct: I'm very relieved. It's out. I've intended to tell you.

Th: I'm so glad you feel relief. What is your sense of how it is for me?

Ct: You seem interested, caring, non-judgmental. I feel very accepted by you.

Th: I'm so glad and also moved by your courage. I feel privileged you've trusted me. I also feel much compassion for your suffering from shame over the years about this secret. How is it for you to hear this from me?

Ct: *(Tears come as he lets in my caring acceptance of forbidden parts of himself. His grief expresses the deprivation he's suffered.)*

We discovered that the only time he saw himself as sexually desirable was when he dressed as a woman. Family members shamed him cruelly as a boy for his sexuality. Without interrupting his defensive storytelling, I could not have held him in his grief and other feelings that emerged.

Find the Courage to be Tenacious

Sharon's anxiety had consumed her for decades after many attempts at therapy. Her words raced, and her tension traveled into my body from emotional contagion.

Ct: After 28 years of marriage and during my bout with cancer, I had the thought of ending my marriage, as my husband was driving me to the hospital for surgery. He'd said he couldn't visit me on the second day until late because the VP of his firm arrived from New Orleans, and he couldn't miss that meeting. My daughter had flown in to be with me, and she needed to spend time with her dad too. I felt like he completely abandoned both of us. So often, I feel alone with him. Even though he's a good provider and a decent man, he's just not there when I need him most.

(The muscles hardened in her jaw, barely perceptible. She then became short of breath and a little dizzy. Her shoulders sagged, and her eyes emptied.)

Th: I see how devastating this experience was for you, and I'm sad you suffered so much. As you told me about this, I saw a fleeting emotion cross your face, and some force seemed to quash it instantaneously. Your energy drained. Did you happen to notice this too? *(She hadn't. By saying, "Did you happen to notice," I imply that I don't assume she would notice. If I ask, "Did you notice?" this subtle difference could evoke shame.)* I know how much you don't want to be anxious, and it looks like your body goes into a fear state when feelings come up (*said with softness and care*). I wonder why there is so little space for your emotions to exist? Do they pose a threat?

Ct: I see no reason to dwell on negative feelings.

Th: Would you want to say what is negative about your feelings?

Ct: I know I have anger at my husband, but that's a useless and terrible feeling. Just look at where that's gotten us in this world!

Th: I agree that acting out anger has wreaked destruction, and neither of us wants any part of that. But here with us, we could make a place for everything you feel, your pure emotions, as they rise in your body, which are a force of nature. Are we to trust nature? If we dismiss your feelings, they will stay submerged and create anxiety. Emotions do not like being ignored.

Ct: I do not want to be anxious, that much I know.

Th: I think that's great. I don't want you to be anxious either. It's a horrible feeling. You've just won half the battle by being willing to recognize that you're angry and being aware that you judge your angry feelings as bad. Would you consider that judgment of your anger causes your anxiety? Might we instead see your anger as valuable? (*Offering an alternative to her self-judgment*).

Ct: I'm willing to try.

She was able to feel sadness for dismissing her feelings throughout her life. But each time she tried to connect to anger toward her husband, massive guilt and shame dominated her effort. In many ways, her husband was a good guy, and she hated her anger, believing she had no right to it. Time and again, she would collapse. Her despair finally got to me. I starkly remember thinking, I give up! I felt vulnerable and began discounting my clinical experience and training. I thought she couldn't do it, and neither could I. It was time to accept that we'd never enter the realm of her unconscious feelings, and I could scramble toward another approach, as I knew a few. Then something told me to dig in for one last final try. Desperation covered Sharon's face.

Th: I feel such sadness for your feelings that never quite make it into the room with us. They try to breathe but are quickly suffocated, never given the gift of life. Some part of you tells them they're evil with no right to exist, and yet you need them, and you suffer so tragically without them. As much as I care, their fate is in your hands. (*I held my breath and prepared for final failure. I honestly saw little future for Sharon's therapy.*)

Ct: I remember when I saw my husband talking to a neighbor across the street, and he looked so much happier, interested, and chatty than he ever is with me. I've tried so hard to reach him, to have even a small bit of that kind of attention. I feel like a powder keg.

Th: Would you be willing to let that energy move through you and give yourself a chance to feel it?

Suddenly she proclaimed her rage impulses toward her husband with clarity, power, and no trace of anxiety! She lifted her head from her hands. Her spine and neck were erect! No trembling! It can't be, I thought. I didn't believe she had it in her to fling the doors open to such freedom of expression. I saw how I'd underestimated both of us. A profound course of treatment ensued, and to our delight, her chronic tormenting anxiety began to evaporate. It's incredible to think that her therapy would have aborted had either of us quit in that session. I wish I could say that I trusted myself and my approach from that day forward, but I fell into doubt countless times, and it was years before I developed steady faith in the therapeutic principles I follow.

What trait do I rely upon most as a therapist? Tenacity. However, tenacity works only with the client's permission and partnership. But what about those times when it's smart to give up and cut our losses? One client told me that a book had convinced her that only a particular form of therapy, which I did not practice, could bring her specific results rapidly. Her belief guaranteed our work would not succeed. I honored her right to her opinion and did not attempt to convince her otherwise. What a striking difference in outcome in these two therapies! Each therapeutic partner has choices to make. When therapists try to carry responsibility for both partners, both will lose. The conscientious therapist reflects on what might have been done differently, but preserving our essential faith in ourselves may be the most important outcome of all. A therapist who had experienced excruciating self-doubts during her training said to me, "I'm so happy because I finally feel I've hit my stride. It was the way you helped me to feel about myself that had the most significant impact."

In therapy, two people take an ancient pilgrimage ever inwards, toward our most profound emotional truths and the origins of the developing self. What journey can be more compelling, enriching and foreboding at the same time? The therapeutic partners attempt to access the most vulnerable, hidden and protected parts within oneself. Sadly, these parts of the self were left by the wayside in the distant past. Someone once bruised or brutalized us, leaving a wreckage of unrepaired ruptures and states of "unbearable aloneness." Our injuries will inevitably become activated in a therapy that reinforces emotional expression. The willingness to bear unresolved emotional pain allows us to move past trauma.

People commonly fear becoming engulfed, trapped or paralyzed by their feelings. They were alone with their feelings at a helpless time in their lives, and that traumatic memory remains. No reference point exists for safely navigating the storms of emotions with a steady other. Research shows that "the more therapists facilitate the affective experience/expression of patients in [a healing relationship], the more patients exhibit positive changes" (Diener et al., 2007, p. 939). Still, our clients wonder, "What unexpected demons will attack me?" "What vile and disgusting parts of me will show themselves?" "Will my therapist see me as pathetic and humiliate me?" "Will I leave my wife if I stay in therapy?" "Will my husband leave me if I grow too much?" "Will I lose my family, my job, my friends?" What courage therapy requires!.

The therapist has opportunities for personal growth in practicing this work too. A well-known teacher told me that his personal therapies had not been particularly helpful, but he'd received the best treatment from practicing psychotherapy. I've changed too through my work. When we sit across from a client and encounter traumas that live in us, there's an eerie familiarity, as we recognize we could be sitting in the client's chair too. I'd ask myself, "How are you going to help someone with similar struggles?" It appeared that I couldn't, but I discovered that both of us could grow simultaneously.

The great David Malan commented, after viewing one of my session videos, "You are fearless." His compliment was lovely. Still, did he know how much uncertainty and self-doubt had assailed me as I worked? Indeed, both therapeutic partners experience fear and dread as they explore the vast unknown. Therapists wonder, "Will my mistakes expose me as an imposter?" "Will my lack of knowledge prove me incompetent?" "Will my client find me lacking?" "Will I know how to handle monstrously big feelings when they surface?" As one trainee said, "I'm afraid I won't be able to handle this degree of emotional intensity hour after hour." Such doubts signal that we're onto something. Didn't we become therapists to work with demons, not avoid them? Of course, being human, we'll try to evade our tormentors. Or we could face our fear, shame, and vulnerability, shining a light of compassion on ourselves and our clients to enter realms we never thought possible.

References

Diener, M. J., Hilsenroth, M. J., & Weinberger, J. (2007). Therapist affect focus and patient outcomes in psychodynamic psychotherapy: A meta-analysis. *American Journal of Psychiatry, 164*(6), 936–941

Knight, J. (1998). *Layers of the ocean: Deep sea creatures on sea and sky.* http://www.seasky.org/deep-sea/ocean-layers.html

Racker, H. (1968). *Transference and countertransference.* International Universities Press.

Tarlow, T.M. (2012). *Clinical intuition in psychotherapy.* W.W. Norton.

2

I DON'T FEEL LIKE FEELING

Our Emotional Rainbow

If a rainbow landed in your backyard, would you assign a value to one hue over another, critiquing and comparing each facet of this shimmering phenomenon? Or would you fall back in awe at this splendorous prism of light? When we encounter our own "emotional rainbow" within ourselves, we typically do not approach our feelings with the wonder they deserve. Instead, we pick apart this rainbow and compartmentalize, minimize, dismiss, condemn, or recoil from its various elements. Fundamental distrust of our emotions is widespread and tragic. When we lose the freedom to feel, marriages fail and families break apart. When we deaden ourselves, we turn to addictions and lose our creative, expressive potential. But of course, it is our life's journey to be lost before we are found.

As forces of nature, feelings have a trajectory and are not subject to our will or beckoning. They simply are. Once activated, they have healthy pathways within our bodies, preordained by nature. Unimpeded, feelings rise to consciousness to be processed, informing our decisions, igniting our creativity, and forging powerful connections to one another. Whether our emotions will "make it home" and fulfill their purpose will

DOI: 10.4324/9780429399633-3

depend on how well we've overcome negative attachment experiences that discourage feelings. The primary obstacles to a non-judgmental awareness of feelings are toxic forms of shame, anxiety, guilt, and self-protective strategies (SAGSS). Whether we find our way out of the thicket of these crushing forces will depend on how much we want to embrace our "emotional rainbow" and free ourselves.

Why would anyone consciously choose to face their emotional pain? Some would view this as masochism. Jed, a middle-aged lawyer, told me that things were going great, his work was extraordinary, and he enjoyed a splendid home in a fashionable area. He said he'd had a brief therapy that didn't help him and added, "The therapist got me to cry a couple of times, and I didn't feel any better afterward. I see no point in dwelling on emotions." He'd recently discovered his wife had an affair. He adored her. We would expect grief and anger, but he reacted with hopelessness and powerlessness. His tears came from a place of depression and despair, and it would have been counterproductive to encourage his weepiness.

A therapeutic trap lurked if I tried to persuade him to "give feelings a chance." Being a professional debater, he had plenty of counter-arguments. If I resisted his resistance, I could set up a futile struggle between him and me. Instead, I reflected on his internal conflict—a man who didn't want to feel chose a "dynamic emotion focused therapist!" In the following exchange from our first session, I focused on clarifying what he wanted from therapy rather than persuading him to feel. Without internal motivation and understanding of the therapeutic process, he'd be likely to drop out of treatment with me too.

Th: What prompted you to call me? (*Desire is the engine of treatment.*)

Ct: I married the love of my life seven years ago. (*She was fifteen years younger than him.*) I thought we were happy, and then she left me abruptly. It broke my heart. She was everything I'd ever dreamed of having in a wife. There was another man. (*His face looked drawn and colorless, as he was devastated by the betrayal. But he didn't say what he hoped to gain from therapy.*)

Th: How painful that must have been!

Ct: It still is. It tore me up. She left for over a year, and I won't say I was a saint during that time. But I never had an interest in anyone else. Now she's come back, and we're seeing a couple's therapist. I'll never be able to know if she'll leave me again.

Th: Yes, I understand. Your trust is terribly damaged. (*I paused, feeling the pathos in his statement and wanting to convey empathy.*) You don't know if you will ever regain a sense of safety in your marriage. (*He expressed his pain with words, but his body seemed detached.*) Tell me more about what you hope to gain from our work? (*Exploring his goals again.*)

Ct: I don't know (*rueful smile*). My wife and our therapist thought I should see someone.

Th: And what do you think?

Ct: I don't see much point in it. (*He wasn't invested in therapy. His body told me so, and we would go nowhere if he weren't onboard.*) I'm happy in every area of my life except for when she left.

He was a proud man who had been humiliated. He defended against his shame and other feelings by letting me know he was successful and high functioning. He denied that he'd been living in a fantasy union and unconsciously contributed to the breakup.

Th: Tell me about why your wife left and why she and your couple's therapist thought you should see an individual therapist? (*Since he saw no internal problem, perhaps his wife might shed some light.*)

Ct: I don't know why they suggested this. (*His wife's primary complaint was that she had "so little sense" of him, just as he had little awareness of the experience of others.*)

Th: For years, you had little idea what she was feeling or vice-versa. This lack of intimacy explains your shock when she left. You've sought my help to please her, but you don't see how therapy can help you. How do you feel about living with this kind of emotional distance in your marriage?

Ct: I'm like most men. Not a feely type.

Th: I get it, but this emotional disconnection led to the biggest disaster in your life, and the pain of loss has been excruciating. I feel sad that you don't wanted more for yourself, and distancing from your wife will keep your marriage on shaky ground. (*Disengagement carries the price of loneliness. I hope to generate compassion for himself.*)

Ct: I'm not unwilling to be in therapy, but I don't know what I can do about it. (*He seems to register that there is a problem within him but feels powerless to change it.*)

Th: Would you want to do something about your emotional detachment if you could (*questioning his will*)? I don't doubt you can feel, but something snuffed it out of you. (*He gets teary.*)

Ct: Yes, I would. I want her to stay. Badly. And I don't want to make her unhappy. I was raised in a very gruff household. My dad expected me to be tough. He was a military guy.

Th: That's a lot of pressure. Yet, I sense your pain, vulnerability, and love, which helps me feel connected to you. And that's what your wife says she wants (*expressing empathy and encouraging his feelings*).

Ct: That's good. It's relieving to know that.

Th: Would you want us to encourage your feelings, as that is the only way to stay connected to your wife and so you will not be a lonely man? (*Helping him to define goals for himself.*)

Ct: I need to do this. I just don't know how.

Th: Do you want to do this?

Ct: Yes. I want to.

Th: Good. I can guide you. We could check in with each other to see how distancing shows up between us (*offering a path creates hope*). We could let each other know when we feel connected and when we don't and how we can increase your sense of safety. When you feel safe, your feelings will find their way. (*The reinforcement of his innate capacity to feel builds confidence that he can change.*) You said that you hadn't felt relief after crying in your last therapy sessions. Feeling your feelings won't stop your pain immediately, but it's the only way to have a relationship with your wife and with yourself as well. I don't think you can know how much your feelings can help you because you have a habit of ignoring them. And sadly, I think you've lost a lot because of this disconnect from yourself.

At the end of this session, he decisively said, "I want to make more appointments." We pulled out our calendars. He stayed in therapy and worked with me far more than I would have imagined, and his marriage improved. What engaged him? It helped to have no expectations of him and to open-endedly explore what he wanted for himself, something he'd never experienced with his family. I made space for him to consider his need for therapy, and he arrived at the following conclusions:

- He wanted his marriage to work.
- He didn't know how to make it work.
- He assumed he could bypass his emotions but realized this wasn't working. His wife had told him she couldn't "sense" him, a major cause of their separation.
- He realized he held a belief that he couldn't work with his feelings productively.
- He saw the possibility to develop his emotional capacities with me.
- He realized he had a choice—to experience and communicate his feelings with my help or risk further alienation from his wife and remain a lonely man.

Seeing that he would have more pain if he continued to avoid his feelings motivated him. An intellectual understanding of this fact would mean little. However, he could feel my sadness for the road that lay ahead of him if he didn't invest in himself, and tears came. It was essential to respect his decision whether to engage in emotion focused therapy. The alliance should never be taken for granted. Although he'd tried to please his wife, he failed because he wasn't emotionally engaged, which could easily happen with us.

Being at peace if a client chooses not to do therapy may be one of the most significant challenges for the therapist. "Am I ok if my client refuses my help?" When I could honestly say, "Yes," my work improved immeasurably. Creating space for Jed to make his decisions was pivotal. He responded by opening up more, telling me that he was defensive and felt afraid and inadequate. When I saw the fear in his eyes, and we could talk about it, I knew we'd made a connection.

Emotional intimacy achieved through a respectful partnership often ushers in remarkable change and recovery. I mention "respectful partnership" because the therapist can use the power of personality to arouse emotional states, which undermines opportunities to build selfhood. Insistent, repetitive questions about feelings often lead to shame responses like, "You want something from me, and I don't know how to give it." Sometimes we insert our will or needs into a session unconsciously, creating pressure on the client to comply. I find it essential to seek permission often, e.g., "Since we know you want to be more able to express your feelings, is it ok with you if we refocus our attention on them?"

Having watched many recorded sessions, I frequently notice phrases like "I need you to ..." or "I want you to ...." When we insert our will, there's a risk. Being directive can reenact trauma associated with domination and humiliation, implying inferiority of the client. We know that repeated suboptimal attachment experiences lead to structural and functional abnormalities in the brain (Newman et al., 2015). In contrast, when we relieve symptoms in psychotherapy, these experiences can alter the brain, creating new connections that disrupt dysfunctional patterns (Cozolino, 2016). Such a quest that reshapes the brain requires the will, courage, and skill to facilitate a deep dive into the vast, formidable, and profoundly curative unconscious world of feelings.

Intuitive, Experiential, and Scientific Support for Emotion Processing

The instant emotions break free, clients describe "relief," "empowerment," and "freedom." One young woman told me, "The fear of showing my emotions just put me in a complete jail." This poignant statement sums up why feelings matter. Research abounds affirming emotion-focused therapy (McCullough & Magill, 2009; Town et al., 2017). Current neuroscientific research indicates that emotional memories must be reactivated and reworked during psychological treatment (Lane et al., 2014), and many studies link in-session affective experience/expression to a positive outcome (Diener et al., 2007). I recollect that Leigh McCullough, Ph.D., found that affective experience at 70% and higher produced the most significant results in her studies. Behavioral change correlated with even 25% emotional activation. Ample evidence argues that the inability to experience complex feelings leads to psychopathology, physical illness, and a host of crippling symptoms (Abbass & Town, 2013; Abbass et al., 2017; Johansson et al., 2014). Therapists instinctively know that working at the highest levels of emotional activation requires skill development. Therapists who work to develop those capabilities are richly rewarded with client satisfaction.

To improve my results, I almost always ask, "How has this session been for you? What has worked? What hasn't been helpful?" Clients invariably rate a session positively that reaches beyond the cognitive mind and unearths emotions. A therapist who said, "I'm looking for something more in my work" yearned for deeper emotional connections with her clients.

Feelings serve as a compass to guide, protect, and provide the inspiration necessary to actualize our lives. Love for my profession compelled me to write this book. Grief honors loved ones we've lost and is essential to recovery. Sexual feelings can awaken a sublime sense of union. Rage can lead to necessary relationship changes. We seek and create art, music, and film because they express our heartfelt passions. Since the avoidance of emotions leads to incalculable suffering, we give the client's feelings the attention they deserve.

Focus on the Most Avoided Emotions

To help our clients focus on their most avoided emotions, we need to recognize them first. Just as children rely upon their parents to help them identify what they feel, our clients depend upon us to help interpret the signals they experience in their bodies. A man says he feels angry, but he experiences an aching pain around his heart, more suggestive of grief. When I point that out, he may recognize that he's defending against the pain of loss and begin to cry. He's likely to be feeling anger too, but we encourage the expression of the feelings that are the most difficult to axxess. Afterwards, we explore what tells him he is angry. (See Figure 2.1 on the physiology of emotion, which provides a valuable guide to identify what the client feels.)

Love

When people can feel their feelings free of shame, guilt, and defense, they won't be in our office. Clients don't need help with what they can feel. They need help with what they can't feel. Gloria, a realtor, wanted relief from high anxiety and sleep disturbance. She sounded harsh, as she vented about the ways her husband had failed her. He was dying in hospice, and she hated going there. She barely spoke to him. Soon her

Physiology of Emotions (with a partial list of examples)	
LOVE, JOY	· Warm sensation · Expansive chest · Desire to touch, embrace, clap, jump
SEXUAL	· Genital arousal · Urge for physical contact
GRIEF, SADNESS	· Heaviness in chest · Ache in heart · Activation around eyes · Urge to weep or sob
FEAR	· Adrenaline rush · Stomach contracts · Sweating · Accelerated heart rate & breathing · Impulse to fight, flee or freeze
ANGER, RAGE	· Striated muscles activated (jaws, shoulders, arms, hands, neck, head, legs) · Aggressive impulse
DISGUST	· Stomach turns, Nausea · Urge to push away
GUILT	· Pain and constriction of the upper chest, larynx, pharynx, and neck muscles · Nausea in the epigastrium

Figure 2.1 Physiology of Emotions.

unmet expectations of him would become final. She was comfortable discharging anger and bitterness. And she became cynical and stubborn when I suggested focusing on her body as a way to relieve her anxiety. She didn't see the point in it and preferred to talk and intellectualize. I accepted her choice after making my best effort. The poignancy of her husband's imminent death struck me. She avoided her tender feelings, which I sensed protected her from her complex feelings around the loss she was facing. After a period of drifting, I circled back to her inaccessible feelings:

Th: I see how painful it is to face the reality that you will never realize your dreams with your husband. You were together over fifty years, which is remarkable, and your children grew into extraordinary, accomplished adults. Was there anything you did find satisfying in your long history together? What attracted you to him?

Ct: He was crazy about me when we met, and he always said we would be married. We had fun and laughed a lot. He had a lot of friends, and I was more inward. We didn't have much in those days, but he would save to take me to dances. I loved to dance! No one ever paid that much attention to me. (*She smiles wistfully.*)

Th: Tell me about other things you appreciated about him.

Ct: We've always had the same values and had a lot in common. Our families were close. He worked extremely hard and provided well for us. I never had to work and had time to be home with my kids. Both of us love our children, and we were both very involved. He keeps telling me to make home repairs, and he worries if I go into unsafe neighborhoods.

Th: He's loved you all these years. Do you sense that he loves you?

Ct: We don't talk about our feelings, but yes, I know he loves me.

Th: What do you feel as we talk about all that you've shared? Are you aware of other feelings besides your anger? (My voice is tender and I pause.)

Ct: It's sad. (*She begins to cry.*) I'm sad for both of us. I'm sad that he's suffering though he doesn't complain. I'll miss him, at least parts of him.

Th: Are you aware of loving feelings for him?

Ct: Yes. I do love Jeff.

Th: I find it tragic that he will not hear the words you have spoken to me. You have pain and anger and terrible loss, and you also have love. I believe it will help both of you to tell him all that you have said to me and all that you recall of your good times together when you visit him. There's not much time left.

She did exactly that in the weeks that followed, even though she felt awkward. Her genuine feelings brought a weak smile to her husband's face. They held hands. Her tears flowed, and she had no regrets about her unspoken love when he passed. She buried him in a beautiful part of Idaho that had meaning to him. She found the setting deeply comforting, and she purchased a lot next to him.

Anger and Rage

The ability to experience anger or rage in the body has motivated people to change laws, fight for causes, and stop abuse or bad treatment. Anger prompts us to address critical issues and can draw us closer to others in the long run. Many consider joy and love to be "positive" while viewing anger as "negative." I don't hold this view. When my clients embrace rage, love deepens, and recovery becomes possible.

Rage has kept me alive. When a suspicious man entered my elevator in downtown San Francisco, I instinctively pushed the 2nd-floor button, even though I was going to the 20th. I was terrified as the door closed. Instantly, he dove under my dress with both arms outstretched. I turned into a human horse, kicking him repeatedly with all my strength and a hammering heart. Thankfully the door opened quickly, and I continued to kick until he fell backward and rolled out of the elevator. I pressed the button to the penthouse floor. Afterwards, the police showed me mug shots and told me he'd escaped from a psychiatric prison and was wanted for raping eleven women in downtown elevators. He was armed and dangerous.

In situations that affect our well-being but are not life-threatening, I never recommend becoming aggressive, pushy, or passive-aggressive, especially if we hope to resolve a difference. Such behavior is guaranteed to alienate or disgust the other person. But when anger merges with anxiety and shame, we're more at risk to act out destructively. Anger triggers retaliatory impulses, but if we inflict pain on others, we'll pay a price in guilt and possible reparations. I want to help my clients experience angry, retaliatory impulses fully within their bodies, recognize the injuries that triggered the anger, and accept their feelings as forces of nature. Imagery facilitates the process. Shame and anxiety drop dramatically once feelings release through the body. The client becomes more relaxed, centered, and freer to explore realistic options. Perhaps the client will address a need more directly or let go of fantasies that someone will change, facing the pain of loss. Maybe we can't recover the love we've lost. But until we let go, we will lose the love we can have today.

Once clients access anger, they may want to express it to the person who wounded them. But many people can't hear anger well, even when communicated respectfully. I wish this weren't true. Unfortunately, people almost always hear anger as criticism and become defensive. I explicitly recommend that my clients self-regulate so they can state their desires in a non-accusatory, non-threatening tone to get a better response.

Some projections need to be cleared up before feelings can be productively explored. For example, if the client is angry at the therapist due to a belief that the therapist dislikes the client or intends harm, we must clarify reality first. If the therapist is viewed as uncaring, the alliance to do deeper work will falter.

A therapist asked, "How do I deal with a client's anger at a partner caused by unrealistic expectations to meet a need that wasn't met in childhood, a loss the person needs to grieve? Do I still explore the anger?" I would explore the anger but only after first addressing the distortion of reality and the splitting defense (i.e., the client disconnects from the good parts of her partner and accentuates the negative).

Ct: I'm furious that he completely forgot that we'd meet at the front entrance to the mall.

Th: I see you were very hurt. Tell me, what does his forgetfulness mean to you?

Ct: If he cared, he wouldn't forget our plans.

Th: So your mind concludes that your husband doesn't care about you. Yet you told me he fought for your care when you were in the hospital. And he took you on a glorious trip for your birthday. You want him to keep track of what you ask of him, but it appears this isn't one of his strengths. When you seek what he can't give, this keeps you in a state of perpetual deprivation. Tell me how you see it (inviting collaboration).

Ct: I know. He can be good to me, and he loves me. It doesn't make sense, but I'm still so mad.

Once she recognizes that her conclusions are distorted, the therapist then returns to the exploration of her anger:

Th: When he appears to dismiss you, anger rises in you and deserves our attention. If we went with the scenario that he stood you up because you're unimportant to him, could we take a look at what this anger feels like in your body? (*This exploration took us back to an early trauma when her mother left her alone for extended periods.*)

Sometimes anger comes from a projection that another person is attacking us, while the self-judgment lies within us. I address projections in the same way I'd treat other distortions of reality. First, clear up the distortion and then explore the underlying feelings to get to the root of the suffering.

Ct: I know he hates me and plans to leave me.

Th: Has he mentioned leaving you?

Ct: No. He's never said anything, and he's home every night, unfortunately.

Th: Might it be possible that the rejection you see in him reflects how you feel about yourself?

Once she can see that there is no evidence that he hates her and plans to leave, explore her initial feelings:

Th: So, we agree we don't know what he's feeling, but your mind creates a scenario. Your feelings about this scenario deserve our attention. If he were plotting to leave you and hated you, how do you feel toward your husband?

Anger and Shame Due to Perfectionistic Ideals

A woman consulted me who had considerable financial resources and was in her late forties, looking fit and ten years younger. After much difficulty with vagueness and unconscious shame, she revealed that her primary concern was that she did not have a partner. Her ex-husband cheated, and a series of disastrous relationships followed, which profoundly discouraged her. She couldn't figure out why years of dating had produced nothing. When I asked what she was looking for in a man, she said, "Someone wealthy and available." Our conversation went like this:

Ct: I went out on a date with a nice man. He has a profession, a stable life, and seems like a decent person. He's smart, and we had fun. We went to a Laguna Beach restaurant, but he parked on the street instead of using the valet. I didn't like that. It's cheap. We then decided to order a large pizza, but he never asked if I wanted anything else. I thought that was rude, only offering me a pizza. (*Her expression conveyed contempt.*)

Th: Did you tell him you wanted to order more?

Ct: I wasn't hungry. I didn't eat that much, and the pizza was filling. But he should have asked if I wanted more.

Th: If you'd said you would appreciate it if he'd offer you more food, what do you think would have happened?

Ct: He probably would have done that, but I didn't want more food. He should have known to ask.

It could be easy to feel disapproval toward her sense of entitlement, but we will see that although her family had wealth, her mother had endured the stinging shame of poverty as a child. Her mother passed on her fears and beliefs that wealth meant belonging and security.

Th: How many men have you met throughout your life who would fulfill your expectations? (*She thinks a long time in silence, but each person who comes to mind has insurmountable flaws. Those whom she idealized were unavailable.*)

Th: Would you agree the evidence tells us the man you seek does not exist (denial in fantasy)? You could keep looking for a perfect man, but what are the odds of finding this type of man you've never met who is without flaws? I also hear that you wish for a man to attune to your desires intuitively without having to reveal your needs explicitly. I'm wondering where this search for an ideal man will take you?

Ct: I'll end up alone and miserable. (*She begins to cry softly.*)

Th: That sounds realistic (*empathically, mirroring her sadness*). So can we say that a highly critical voice inside you demands an impossible standard and keeps you miserable? (*This comment shifts the focus from an external problem (there are no good men) to an internal, workable problem (her judging mind, harsh standards and avoidance of underlying feelings.*)

Ct: Nitpicky. I'm a bitch.

Th: Do you think we could look at this problem honestly without judging you? Perhaps we could look at the feelings that lie beneath your contempt for the men you meet?

Ct: Yes. (*She sighs deeply as feelings are activated.*)

Th: What did you feel toward this man when he didn't ask if you wanted more than a pizza?

Ct: Annoyed. (*This was the first time she'd admitted any degree of anger.*)

Th: Yes, good you could recognize that! You had some degree of anger. Some internal force rapidly submerges this feeling and takes you to your default place, which is to withdraw. This learned habit pushes your anger and your relationships off a cliff. Would you agree? (*I have intentionally referenced an internal force rather than using a "you" message—"You submerge your feelings"—as "you" points a finger and evokes shame and fails to acknowledge unconscious "not me" forces.*)

Ct: Yes. That's what happens precisely! Everything goes off a cliff.

Th: Most unfortunately, this habit keeps you alone. Do you agree? (*With sadness in my voice.*)

Ct: Yes (*becoming tearful*). I've never been able to sustain a relationship.

Th: You've been programmed to have a judging mind that concludes that no man is good enough, and you as a failure for not finding a flawless partner. When you encounter shortcomings, you despair and withdraw, and there is no room to work through your feelings or your conflicts. We could say you maintain optimal distance. Either you attach to a man who will leave you, or, if he is available, you will withdraw.

Ct: Right. I give up. I don't know what I feel. And I don't tell men what I need. (*She revealed her self-doubts, social anxieties, and history of anorexia.*)

Th: It's tragic that an internal force discounts your feelings and harms you, perhaps more than any man has done.

Ct: So, what can be done? (*She becomes tearful.*)

Th: Could we make some space for your sadness first? Your tears matter. (*Her tears flow. I wait until they subside.*) There's an alternative (*said with tenderness*). Would you want us to help you break free of your dominating, judging mind so you can become more tolerant of yourself and others? Would you want to make room for human deficits and work through your feelings so you can sustain a relationship?

Ct: I didn't realize it had to be one or the other (*work through feelings or remain alone*).

Th: It does. (A clear, unambiguous message helps.)

Ct: I want to do this. I need to do this.

Th: Good! I'd love to help you to take notice of your feelings and begin to value them. I believe you will discover more happiness.

She reflects on her parents' absolute certainty about their opinions and superiority and how they caused her to feel perpetually inadequate. She realized their lives were far from perfect, and she began to look at the impact her idealization of them had on her life. Seeing this reality was a breakthrough moment. She'd been seeking perfection in the men she dated and in herself because of the unrealistic fantasies her parents created. We would need to explore her complex feelings toward them.

Grief Blocked by Guilt

Experiencing grief is necessary to heal from losses. Brenda told me she'd abruptly lost her soulmate after 30 years of marriage. She wasn't sure if she needed therapy. She'd grieved on occasion since her husband's death, but mostly she kept constantly busy. She'd sold their properties and relocated, and she had an active social and family life. Her busyness avoided her grief and other feelings. She appeared anxious and guarded, making furtive eye contact, which telegraphed her shame. She said she'd had several courses of therapy, repeatedly assuring me how well she was functioning. She downplayed her needs or suffering, which had caused her to contact me.

When I inquired into the details of her husband's death, she looked down. A downward glance can mean a lot of things. As we talked in detail about her husband's medical treatment, the question arose within me, "Could I have done more in that terrible situation?" Perhaps she had that question too. Following my instincts, I asked her gently if it might be possible that she was carrying guilt about his death? Conveying compassion is essential to open doors to new exploration. She seemed shocked at the word, and pain flashed across her face. She disclosed that she hadn't been as active in his health care as she could have been. Maybe she could have done more to save him. She hadn't been involved in his choice of doctors and wasn't aware he had some bad drug reactions. She immediately recognized that "guilt" named her true feeling, which had gone unrecognized for a long time. She expressed pain and relief to have brought her guilt into the open. She said this feeling was never discussed in her prior therapy. In reality, she had played a role in the fact that her beloved husband had received inadequate care. How awful to face! I encouraged her to take some time to feel her pain and remorse. She cried.

Brenda looked down as she mentioned enjoying her new home on the lake, saying that her husband wouldn't have chosen it. I asked if being happy in the house that he could not enjoy and would not have chosen added to her guilt? She said, "Yes!" We needed to differentiate her toxic survivor's guilt, related to her new life, from necessary remorse for those times she overlooked her husband's needs. Her busyness suggests that she avoids grieving, reflecting, and dealing with her guilt, preventing her from enjoying the positive parts of her life. Her busyness may also have made her less aware and available when her husband needed her. In the sessions to follow, she said that discovering her guilt had been a revelation, and she was feeling lighter. Therapists often overlook guilt in treatment—yet healthy and toxic forms of guilt are vital to distinguish and uncover.

Consequences of Inhibiting the Feeling of Rage

In the following case, a woman has repressed anger at her father, resulting in symptoms of anxiety and depression:

Th: Rageful impulses are inside you, but they've been rejected and pushed out of your awareness. I have similar feelings within myself (*normalizing rage*) and appreciate my anger at times—especially when I'm threatened or wounded.

Ct: I'm glad I'm not the only one. I see the value.

Th: Imagine not having anxiety or depression as your constant companions, not biting your lips or having balls of heat knotted up in your chest. Not getting depressed. Feeling your rage does not harm your father. Nobody's getting hurt except you.

Ct: I guess I'm just afraid. It feels like I'm playing with a grenade. I'm scared that one day I'll have some intense anger at somebody and just snap.

Th: Like your dad beat up on you. Another option is you could feel rage without acting on it, unlike your dad. We can just notice how this anger is showing up in your body. I hear your fear. (*Repeating the word "rage" increases exposure to this avoided emotion.*)

Ct: I'm trying to put it in terms that I can relate to. I guess. (*She thinks for a moment, and nods her head as if to say, "Yes, I got it."*)

Th: Tell me what helps you to relate to this possibility of feeling rather than acting on your rage?

Ct: Knife safety in a restaurant. (*She's an expert chef.*) To avoid cutting yourself, the proper way to hold your knife in relation to the hand that's holding the food is that the knife should be right up against your knuckles. That's one of the hardest things I have to teach any students because they're so afraid of cutting themselves that they don't want to put their hands near the knife. But what butting the knife up against your knuckles does is provides a guard for your fingertips, and it also lets you know exactly where the knife is in relation to your hands at all times, so there's no chance of you cutting yourself.

Th: Great metaphor!

Ct: That's how I'm relating to this. I can't be afraid of the knife.

Th: Right. And when you're aware of the knife, you can be sure it doesn't hurt you. That's a marvelous analogy.

Are Some Feelings Better than Others?

Most people think so, yet every emotion we experience arrives with us at birth in a latent form. No feelings are accidents of nature. Dysregulated feelings wreak havoc on our bodies, but regulated feelings serve as signals that guide us away from pain and toward the satisfaction of our needs. Our pleasures become more selfless as we mature. Only when our feelings fulfill their purpose do they exit naturally, of their own accord.

People often harshly judge their feelings. I wish to put all feelings on an equal footing and offer my clients an understanding of their context. I encourage my clients to value their feelings and tend to them with a spacious, welcoming acceptance, a radically new perspective for most people. Feelings are often categorized into primary and secondary states, as some emotions trigger others. Still, while grief may follow rage, does that make grief more important to experience than rage? If I were to give more importance to any emotion, it would be the emotion a client avoids, fears, or causes shame. Let's say a woman is weepy. Although I know complex feelings are present, I want to first acknowledge her sadness, and then encourage the feelings that she finds hard to reach. I may say, "I see you're in pain. Let your tears come." Sometimes tears express anxiety alongside other feelings. "Do you have a sense of other feelings besides your sadness?" Emotions are non-linear, non-hierarchical, overlapping, and part of a complex neurobiological system.

I'll never forget a man dying of cancer. He said, "It's my pain, and it belongs to me. No one can take it away from me." He was right. He didn't want anyone to dismiss his painful feelings to help themselves to feel better. His suffering was part of his life experience, and he wished to own its importance. People commonly want to keep some emotions and dump others. But it doesn't work well that way. If we're going to feel our feelings, we need to give equal attention and space to the "bad" ones. Paradoxically, this makes the "good" ones fuller.

Tragically, a young woman with a history of sexual abuse had learned to ignore what she felt:

Ct: Why is this still a problem? These assaults happened a long time ago. My older sister advised me not to tell my father that his brother molested me because it would kill him. So I didn't, and I pushed it out of my mind. I thought it was behind me, yet I'm having recurring nightmares that have remnants of that experience.

Th: Your uncle perpetrated a crime upon you that continues to torment you because your feelings are trapped. Our emotions are like children, forces of nature that knock at the door of our awareness. We don't get to pick and choose our feelings. They simply are. They want to be heard and witnessed. What will happen when you turn your back on children knocking at your door?

Ct: They'll probably get frustrated.

Th: Will they go quietly into the night?

Ct: No, they will knock harder.

Th: Yes. Do we provide your feelings with an audience, or do we reject them and drive them into nightmarish forms?

Ct: I don't want to turn away from them.

There are only two possibilities. Feelings, desires, impulses, and sensations will rise to awareness and receive caring attention, or judgment and fear will drive them into our interior and reshape them into unrecognizable and punishing forms.

Th: Wow! So, if you and I invite your feelings into this room, feelings that are natural forces rising in your body—like a snowstorm, torrential rainfall, or the sun—your emotions will bring down destruction and devastation to all you love?

Ct: Yes. I believe that.

Th: And yet there is no one here but you and me. Your dad is probably on the golf course at this very moment, and your mom is having lunch with her friends. They will go on with their lives after our session ends, will they not?

Ct: Yes. It does seem rather silly.

Th: But what happens to you? You will continue to suffer from debilitating depression. I believe these feelings come to us as gifts, as friends. Sadly you've learned to shun them, which is like being ashamed of the molecules in the rain. How is it for you to hear me describe feelings in this way?

Ct: Very cool and compelling, like moving toward freedom of expression, uncensored.

When we can embrace rather than judge these feeling life forces within us, visceral and profound insights often emerge. As a teenager, an addict had plotted to kill his father after he violently beat his mother. When his rage first bubbled to the surface in a session, he jumped out of his chair. I'd never had this experience before or since. (See Pete vignette, Chapter 6, for more details.) Fear overcame him, and he said, "I don't want you close to my anger." Once his rage could break through multiple times, he told me that he'd stopped obsessing about his father and rarely thought about him anymore. When he did, he noticed a new feeling of softness toward him, and he was able to recall positive memories of him.

Countless times I've seen people rekindle loving feelings after they have passed through the unlikely doorway of violent rage impulses, an energy current the body can feel. The hands may form fists, or heat rises in the chest. We track the rage impulses as they naturally move to the outer extremities. We utilize fantasy to imagine the release of these impulses as they leave the body and fully express themselves, like a wild animal. The client may notice an urge to pound or grab while sitting in the chair and harming no one. The client and therapist observe and share. That's it! An anger-phobic client said to me, "I got a call at my job, and this fury exploded within me, and I took a walk and let myself feel it. The impulses came like a torrent, wave after wave, very intense. But then they burned themselves out. They didn't stick around. I was able to return to my work." She couldn't believe that anger would move on when she allowed herself to feel it. One emotion leads to others, and when all are accepted an old adage come alive, "The truth shall set you free." But it is more than truth. It is a truth that can be shared within a caring relationship that sets us free.

The power of such a process is very different from catharsis, discharge, or acting out. Such states indicate that excessive anxiety, shame, or guilt have dysregulated the nervous system to the point of losing control and potentially doing harm to self or others (McCullough Vaillant, 1997). My client was over the threshold for anxiety tolerance when he jumped out of the chair. I immediately and soothingly encouraged him to return to his chair, so we could connect again and immediately regulate his anxiety, allowing him to tolerate his feelings.

In another case, an adult son hurled accusations of failure and incompetent parenting at his father. His loud and aggressive discharge caused excruciating pain for his father and triggered guilt in the son, which fueled his depression. Were the son able to deal with his anger in a more regulated state, it would be far more productive for both. An astute clinician, who had watched me deal with a client's rage in a fantasy, worried that I might encourage acting out in real life. It's just the opposite. I would steadfastly discourage acting out while reinforcing the safe processing of rage as an internal experience that is shared in my office.

Therapists can unknowingly encourage dysregulated states. A therapist described a session with a client who was regressing to a traumatized state. The young man crawled under a table, and the therapist crawled after him and began conversing with him in a huddled position for some time. In another instance, the client asked to lie down for most of the session, not due to any illness. The therapist agreed without any exploration. Reinforcing these regressive states underestimates the capacity of the client. A sense of mastery is a common factor that leads to therapeutic change (Weinberger, 1995). Across all models, a sense of mastery involves helping the client to face and conquer fears and tolerate new emotional states. When the therapist and client together provide sufficient regulation, involving continual monitoring of bodily sensations with caring and reflection, the client can gradually bear the far reaches of the emotional underworld. "Surviving an emotionally intense experience can directly strengthen patients' self-confidence and mastery. Such an experience may also encourage patients to enter into and cope successfully with situations they previously feared or avoided, further bolstering their morale" (Frank & Frank, 1993). Both the therapist and client must build the capacity to stay present to all experiences, eyes wide open. These higher states of consciousness are modeled by master meditators who resist nothing, making deep integration possible.

Enhanced self-acceptance is a manifestation of love. People have a hard time seeing themselves as a person worthy of love because we're inside ourselves! Yet, we need to embrace ourselves to embrace others. What greater cruelty than to ignore or loathe oneself? And how can a person progress in therapy without dissolving the shame and fear that prevents us from knowing ourselves? True love is neither blind nor naive. Love sees the cracks and wraps its arms around the broken parts within us. Love is the bedrock for growth.

We cannot love without first being loved. Humans yearn to feel safe in a relationship above all else, though these longings may be unconscious and fervently denied. The therapist offers an emotional presence that can hold all parts of the self, without risk of judgment or withdrawal. When such an encounter is real and rich in quality, some call it love.

> Our patients arrive in our consulting rooms wondering, 'Can you help me?' If therapy progresses and the relationship deepens as risks are

> taken and the heart becomes more vulnerable, a second question, whether spoken aloud or not, arises: 'Do you love me?' The degree to which our patients reveal what they have so vehemently defended against, and often despised about themselves, is the degree to which they consciously or unconsciously hope that we will love them—for who they are, as well as for who they are not. (Quillman, 2020)

My fondest hope is that through our journey together, my clients will walk away able to answer that question, "Did she love me?" Yes.

> "Love is not love
> Which alters when it alteration finds,
> Or bends with the remover to remove:
> O no; it is an ever-fixed mark,
> That looks on tempests, and is never shaken."
>
> (Shakespeare, 1609)

References

Abbass, A. A., & Town, J. M. (2013). Key clinical processes in intensive short-term dynamic psychotherapy. *Psychotherapy*, 50(3), 433–437. https://doi.org/10.1037/a0032166

Abbass, A., Town, J., Ogrodniczuk, J., Joffres, M., & Lilliengren, P. (2017). Intensive short-term dynamic psychotherapy trial therapy: Effectiveness and role of "unlocking the unconscious". *Journal of Nervous and Mental Disease*, 205(6), 453–457. https://doi.org/10.1097/NMD.0000000000000684

Cozolino, L. J. (2016). *Why therapy works: Using our minds to change our brains*. W.W. Norton.

Diener, M. J., Hilsenroth, M. J., & Weinberger, J. (2007). Therapist affect focus and patient outcomes in psychodynamic psychotherapy: A meta-analysis. *The American Journal of Psychiatry*, 164(6), 936–941. https://doi.org/10.1176/appi.ajp.164.6.936

Frank, J. D., & Frank, J. B. (1993). *Persuasion and healing: A comparative study of psychotherapy*. Johns Hopkins University Press.

Johansson, R., Town, J. M., & Abbass, A. (2014). Davanloo's intensive short-term dynamic psychotherapy in a tertiary psychotherapy service: Overall effectiveness and association between unlocking the unconscious and outcome. *PeerJ*, 2, e548. https://doi.org/10.7717/peerj.548

Lane, R. D., Ryan, L., Nadel, L., & Greenberg, L. (2014). Memory reconsolidation, emotional arousal, and the process of change in psychotherapy: New insights from brain science. *Behavioral and Brain Sciences, 38*, E1. https://doi.org/10.1017/S0140525X14000041

McCullough, L., & Magill, M. (2009). Affect-focused short-term dynamic therapy. In R. A. Levy & J. S. Ablon (Eds.), *Handbook of evidence-based psychodynamic psychotherapy: Bridging the gap between science and practice* (pp. 249–277). Humana Press. https://doi.org/10.1007/978-1-59745-444-5_11

McCullough Vaillant, L. (1997). *Changing character: Short-term anxiety-regulating psychotherapy for restructuring defenses, affects, and attachment.* Basic Books.

Newman, L., Sivaratnam, C., & Komiti, A. (2015). Attachment and early brain development – Neuroprotective interventions in infant–caregiver therapy. *Translational Developmental Psychiatry, 3*(1), 28647. https://doi.org/10.3402/tdp.v3.28647

Shakespeare, William (1936). Sonnet 116. In T. Brooke (Ed.), *Shakespeare's sonnets.* Oxford University Press. (Original 1609).

Town, J. M., Salvadori, A., Falkenström, F., Bradley, S., & Hardy, G. (2017). Is affect experiencing therapeutic in major depressive disorder? Examining associations between affect experiencing and changes to the alliance and outcome in intensive short-term dynamic psychotherapy. *Psychotherapy, 54*(2), 148–158. https://doi.org/10.1037/pst0000108

Quillman, Trip (2020) Neuroscience and the therapist's love for the patient: Intersubjective space, the embodied imagination, and transformation. *Journal of Spirituality in Mental Health, 22*(1), 1–29. https://doi.org/10.1176/appi.psychotherapy.1996.50.1.14

Weinberger, J. (1995). Common factors aren't so common: The common factors dilemma. *Clinical Psychology: Science and Practice, 2*(1), 45–69. https://doi.org/10.1111/j.1468-2850.1995.tb00024.x

3

DESIRE IS THE ENGINE OF TREATMENT

Bringing Goals into Focus

Hope is not an endpoint but rather a dynamic process that initiates and propels therapeutic movement. Researchers widely recognize hope as a primary agent for psychotherapeutic change across various theoretical approaches (Larsen & Stege, 2010), so therapists do well to take the pulse of hope throughout treatment. May we grow keenly aware of the therapeutic elements that give birth to hope and ignite the psychic energy to promote transformation. Experience taught me to direct attention immediately to discouragement with the therapeutic process, as waning hope is a crucial indicator of disengagement from therapy.

Hope and desire fuel the engine of treatment, and they are inextricable. Bringing desires into sharp focus catalyzes change, but goals must be attainable. Yearning without a realistic expectation for fulfillment leads to despair. Hope grows stronger when our clients grasp how we propose to work together as a team to arrive at their chosen destinations. We engender confidence when we convey that we know the route well, have had many past successes with similar problems, and will not

DOI: 10.4324/9780429399633-4

abandon the client when the going gets tough. It's crucial that the client sees the therapist as a trusted, competent ally. Outcome studies show that therapy is more effective when patients feel hopeful about specific therapeutic processes (Frank & Frank, 1993; Imber et al., 1970; Wilkins, 1979).

The path we recommend to our clients involves both therapy partners giving caring attention to all internal experiences including the following:

1 Bodily sensations
2 Rising feelings
3 Thoughts and beliefs that impact the process
4 Noticing how well the relationship is functioning

Are the therapeutic partners feeling connected and taking risks together? The therapist and client need to co-regulate their relationship, as the client will go nowhere when feeling alone or misunderstood. I told a couple how much I rely on their feedback to serve them well. They appreciated my comment. This focused partnership helps the client sustain regulated states and move beyond treatment obstacles, making it possible to explore one's feelings more freely. Offering a defined path generates hope. We assure the client that we've successfully taken this journey many times before. We're familiar with the obstacles and how to surmount them through a joint effort. We'll be alongside our clients every step of the way, and we will not desert them as long they desire our help. "Hope is the greatest gift we can offer our clients" (Berg & Dolan, 2001).

What is a Visceral Vision?

Effective goals are desires that live in the body. We might call them visceral visions. Some of my favorite synonyms for "visceral" are: intuitive, instinctual, internal, interior, abdominal, inborn, and rooted. The part about "abdominal" intrigues me, as I hold states of intention in my belly. When I focus on a goal, energy activates in my core. As I observe this phenomenon, I associate to the phrases "girding the loins," "generative power," "preparing oneself for action," and "fire in the belly," which has been described as "the emotional stamina and vigor, passion, or inner drive to achieve something, to take action."

The following vignette with Hannah illustrates her "visceral vision," a deeply felt desire that reaches beyond cognition. Her body registered feelings about what she wanted in the future and wanted to leave behind from the past. I drew attention to her numbing shame, which led to a desire for freedom from the internal bully that flattened her life force. Hannah's "visceral vision" stirred energy in her body, and when she felt hope, her chest and arms expanded, her face broke into a smile, and her breathing became freer. Hannah also wanted to release her primitive projections that others looked down on her so she could refocus her energies on productive goals. She described a new desire emerging:

Ct: I had a different relationship to my will all of a sudden. I've always thought of will as muscling it or creature-powering things until I can't hold it anymore, and then I blow. And I finally connected to this adult woman's will in me that was very different. It was like I wanted it. I want it, as opposed to feeling it's something externally imposed on me. And that was new.

Th: Ah. Wonderful! What did you want?

Ct: Wanting to be an adult woman, like really live in that place, no longer animate the stuff over here that discounts me and destroys everything that I've built.

Th: So you don't want to fall into a bottomless pit of shame and passivity due to forces that undo your efforts?

Ct: Yes! When I got in touch with that will and the reality that my torment is not going to disappear magically, then I want to build something else. I want to do the work that I need to do to sustain something else. And that felt grounded, really solid. I experience it as a woman deep within me, feminine and very powerful. And I feel her in my solar plexus. Deep in there. She's not stubborn, but she's grounded.

Th: So, you want to live in a place that's not at the mercy of fear and shame and being out of control. You feel this grounded desire in your solar plexus. How do you envision going forward from the lost state to the found state? (*She smiles.*)

Ct: Someone said something this week that I could take personally, and I'd typically become very combative, and I could get a lot of mileage out of it. But this week, I resisted those impulses three times with different people. It's just not productive. If I'm going to stabilize the adult and grow that ability, I need not take things personally and be this flighty, reactive, insecure person.

Th: So, you'd like us to continue working together to strengthen the adult woman in you, a woman who stays connected to her desires and feelings and is not at the mercy of shaming internal forces or irrelevant external forces? (*Defining her goals.*)

Ct: Yes! Precisely! I feel energy now.

Th: Tell me how the energy feels in your body?

Ct: It feels good. I can breathe better (*big smile*). Plenty of energy to do whatever I need to do. It's coming up. I feel a lot in my solar plexus. Recently I was able to write a song after a period of being blocked, and I also had the energy to organize my workspace. Now I feel embarrassed. (*I intuit that she projects that I disapprove of her as she reveals progress and competence. Many clients have been humiliated for drawing positive attention to themselves.*)

Th: How do you experience me as you expose this powerful, energetic, creative you? (*My question seems to jar a realization about her distorted perception of me, and she suddenly sees me as I am.*)

Ct: I like you more and more. A lot. And then I like the colors of you, like the aqua of your shirt, the red of your hair and the color of your lips. Then you're somebody there to play with, engage with, and go like, "Isn't life cool?" Aren't people bizarre and wacky (*she laughs*)? Like we have this secret about life and people.

Th: Tell me more about your experience of us.

Ct: I feel it as this alive, wild but fun, wise energy. I feel that in you. And if I can experience that in you, then I can experience that in me, and it's enjoyable.

Th: Beautiful! (*I appreciate her sense of safety and freedom.*)

Ct: And what we could do, the fun we could have, the relationship, the trouble we could get into. (*Both of us giggle in delight.*) There's nothing we couldn't handle, not blinded by anything, not naive.

Th: How is it to share this with me? (*Checking in frequently as the client reveals more is vital.*)

Ct: It's scary. It's hard to get over being seen, being embarrassed to be seen.

Th: If the shame force had dominated today and we had denied ourselves this spirit of celebration, what a loss for both of us!

Shame often inhibits the expression of "I want," or "I desire," or "I feel." This woman's desires are viscerally felt in her body. By contrast, she experiences how shame drains energy from her body, restricting her breathing, and aggravating a stomach disorder. Later in the session, she expressed anger toward her shame and then observed:

Ct: Even how I'm saying that now, "We're not going to go there anymore," I'm having trouble moving my mouth. That's the thing! (*She notices her slowed speech and throws her hands into the air, smiling broadly upwards.*) Ahhh!! There's the energy, and that's what creates the conflict. (*She demonstrates her slow-speed voice and her normal voice.*) Instead of being in my body, speaking, moving, alive—(*She throws her arms in the air again and makes punctuation marks with her hands to show the contrast.*)

Th: It's wonderfully freeing to feel everything and to feel safe in a relationship.

I'm pleased as Hannah defines her wish to step confidently and freely into the world in the early sessions. She's aware of her internal conflicts, which manifest physiologically—the shame that makes her powerless and slows her speech, and the hope and desire that allow her to expand. She recognizes she can make a choice. Being able to experience her range of expression gives her hope. Several studies find that "the best predictor of later benefits is … [the expectation] of early benefits expressed in the early sessions" (Luborsky 1976). Hope is understood to play a pivotal role in early psychotherapy sessions, i.e., 3–4 weeks (Horvath & Greenberg, 1994; Ilardi & Craighead, 1994; Wickramasekera, 1985; Wilkins, 1979, 1985).

For years I held sessions where neither the client nor I were clear about treatment goals. Were we making progress and were the client's desires for treatment waxing or waning? Sometimes in supervision, therapists will draw a blank when I ask, "What does the client want now?" We don't need to ask this question compulsively. But periodically, we need to clarify the client's desires and see if the engine of treatment is turned on or idling. Amazing things happen when clients commit to specific goals or desires. Yet there are exceptions. Some clients experience their goals as "authoritarian dictators …" and "pressing the issue may decrease rapport …" (Bresler & Starr, 2015). Might some clients experience their goals as authoritarian dictators due to shame, impossible standards, and compliance with others' expectations? In my experience, when clients tap into their goals from a deeply authentic and realistic place, their goals become a way to honor themselves. It helps to explore multiple goals in the first session and notice emerging, new goals throughout treatment. When we create an evolving "hope portfolio" with multiple objectives, all hope is not lost when one goal hasn't been realized (Larsen & Stege, 2010).

Goals may be actualized in one moment and abandoned in the next or replaced by something entirely different. They travel from foreground to background in treatment and can serve the good or not so good. Goals that are grounded in unrealistic fantasy breeds despair. Hope or lack of hope operates implicitly or explicitly and impacts the direction of therapy. A direct inquiry is often necessary to bring the state of hope to our awareness. Affirmative and clarifying responses to any of these questions breed hope.

"What are you hoping for today?"

"Do you see progress toward your goals today?"

"What hopes have been satisfied in your therapy since we began?"

"Have you reached for goals in your life and achieved them?"

"Do your old achievements give you hope for new ones?"

The therapeutic journey requires fluidity, freedom, mystery, experimentation, and curiosity. The client and therapist co-create a tapestry, not knowing what the finished art will look like precisely or whether the threads will be wool, gold, or silver. The outcome may surprise us! Still, we want to know, "What are we working toward?" and "Are we moving forward?" "What new visions are emerging?" "What is working and what isn't?" Only our clients can know for sure, and hopefully, they will tell us! And we can ask.

In *The Act of Creation*, Arthur Koestler wrote about scientific and artistic geniuses who made civilization-shaping discoveries while musing in a bathtub or awakening from a dream state. These epiphanies were not isolated incidents. Rather, they evolved after these individuals had pursued particular answers and solutions during years of study and experimentation (Koestler, 1964). Their passionate desires to create or discover something new fueled this process. In therapy, body-based desires are critical to those eventual breakthroughs.

The Language of Desire

"I want freedom from my terrors." "I want to feel trust without dread so that I might remarry one day." "I want the courage to finish my book." "I want to feel more of the safety that I feel with you right now." "I like it when my shoulders drop. My body wants to feel like this more often." If we intend to treat such desires seriously, don't we need to keep track of them? If they evaporate from consciousness, will we harness their power in therapy? Therapists may need to take notes to remember the client's exact words describing their desires as they evolve through treatment. I often reference the client's desires precisely to activate the will to take greater emotional risks.

When we focus on the client's desires, we communicate, "Your longings matter to me." This message builds selfhood. If we predetermine the direction of therapy, we show a lack of faith in the client's capacity to set goals. When we see a client struggling with a sense of direction, we may think we need to take over. But shortcuts come with a price. Instead, we can help the client explore the cost of passivity regarding one's needs: "It looks like you've come to therapy for your wife. What happens to your voice and your wishes? I wonder if your desires have taken a back seat at other times in your life?" Is it important for you to have your feelings considered?" When we direct the client, we dominate rather than empower. Selfhood comes from exercising autonomy, taking risks, gaining mastery, and feeling safe in the process.

Exposing Needs and Desires Trigger Shame

When we inquire about personal goals, we may miss the shame, anxiety, guilt, and self-protective responses that such exploration often evokes. Or, we may retreat from clarifying goals to avoid increasing the client's discomfort. Rather than push a client to set goals or abandon the effort, we can express empathy for the person's difficulty defining deeply felt desires. For example:

Th: When I ask what you hope for in our work together, you seem to become uncomfortable. Am I perceiving this accurately?

Ct: I suppose. I don't think about myself that much. I don't have a clear idea.

Th: Maybe someone made you feel ashamed of giving this kind of attention to yourself, so it's hard to name what you want for yourself?

Ct: That sounds right.

Th: How unfortunate that giving attention to your desires was discouraged. But if we step into this new territory, we could help you clarify what you aim for in therapy, and you'll be more satisfied with the outcome. Would you want us to try to gain more clarity?

Therapists can meet unconscious needs in therapy without articulating them. But if needs have no name, and the client doesn't know how to pursue their fulfillment, how does the client gain more satisfaction in their outside lives? When our clients learn to attend consciously to their wants and desires, they have a far better chance of finding fulfillment. Once needs are declared, unexpected solutions to problems and sources of support may arrive through no conscious effort. Recognizing internal barriers to feelings, aspirations, and desires sets in motion a healing process, as we'll see in the following example. This client's ex-husband had had a long-standing affair:

Ct: It's hard for me to ask for what I want.

Th: I see. That probably would have led to tolerating deprivation in your marriage?

Ct: I would agree with that. And also feeling neglected. Um, feeling—

Th: Neglected by? (*I ask her to specify the source of neglect.*)

Ct: Like betrayed, or I'm not worth anything. Everything else comes before me on his checklist and mine. (*She laughs.*)

Th: That's a great observation. Both of you dismiss your needs, and you have feelings about that. That seems so sad, but there's laughter.

Ct: That's really true. I do dismiss myself. (*She looks down as sadness rises.*)

Th: Although we can't control your husband's habits, do we both agree that your practice of treating your desires as unimportant has caused you suffering?

Ct: Unfortunately, yes.

Th: Earlier, you said you want to reclaim your life and find yourself, which is something entirely new, right? (*She agrees.*) You want us to show more caring attention toward you and your feelings. Is that right?

Ct: Yeah, I would agree. And I'm terrified.

Excellent! She has identified her fear of her feelings and her desires. We began to explore anxiety in her body. She was short of breath, her heart pounded, and she couldn't think clearly. Her anxiety rose due to a projection onto me that I would attack her for declaring her desires and feelings. In the past, her mom had erupted with rage when she said what she needed. She found it profoundly healing to discover we could forge a new relationship together.

New Emotional Freedoms Unleash New Desires

Goals can shift rapidly in treatment as people grow. As the client's self-care grew stronger, she envisioned being with a caring partner after years of being alone. But then she thought, "What makes me think I can have something I've never known?" My fear of heights wouldn't allow me to desire to climb K2. Pursuing desires successfully requires a psychological structure. "Can I face my human limitations and set goals that are attainable?" "Can I bear the loss if I declare my dreams and they don't come to fruition? If I audition for this part and don't get it, will I allow rejection to define who I am?" When we no longer project that our flaws will make us undesirable to others, we won't feel so frightened. When our clients discover we won't leave or judge them, they can risk more.

A woman who was tormented by suicidal ideation and anger turned against herself made the following comments:

"It was very relieving to me to share my feelings about the sexual shaming I'd had as a child and the promiscuous behavior that resulted from it. I'd told only one other person in my life about this. I want this kind of openness with my family too." "It was so hard to talk to you about betraying my best friend because I felt ashamed and guilty. Yet I felt great relief. Other things I've done in the past have haunted me, and so I want to get these things off my chest, too."

She deeply sighed as she brought her transgressions into the open, and I felt like a mother confessor. Waves of painful guilt moved through her, followed by relief that made her more determined to resolve every incident of doing significant harm to another. This painful path was riddled with thorns, but we found ways to experience compassion for those she'd injured and also for her need for primitive defenses. She didn't want to leave a stone unturned from her buried past. She was not storytelling. She released grief at the horrors of her actions. No repairs were possible because the people she'd hurt had died or were no longer reachable. But she became clear she would not betray or violate others or herself again. This emergent goal allowed her to move beyond her self-hatred and shame to feel worthy of being in a relationship with others. She became transparent and authentic with her grown children to a degree she had never before experienced.

Daring to Reach for More

Envisioning new possibilities activates impulses to seek, but trauma exerts a powerful pull to retreat. Early experiences wire our brains to expect the future to repeat the past. "If I become more real or transparent, will my husband still want me? Or will he abandon me as my father did?" "If I speak up about my preferences, will people see me as self-centered, as my mother did?" The traumatized mind links present desire to past rejection, so defenses drive desires into the unconscious. Helping our clients give voice to latent yearnings sets wheels in motion that have a life of their own. I'm often asked: "So how did you go so deep into feelings in the first sessions?" The power of desire is a driving force. Hannah declared her wish to tap into her robust, expressive adult woman but reaching this goal required us to deactivate her shame and regulate her anxiety, which were aroused when she revealed her hidden longings.

The work requires that the client's desires for therapy become conscious. As we descend into the deeper realms of emotional intimacy, formidable barriers inevitably block our path. When I attempted to explore a distancing pattern with a client, she perceived me as attacking her. Knowing that she sought therapy to sustain a relationship and feared a life alone, I could more effectively intervene. Her vulnerable disclosure allowed me to draw attention to the ways she unconsciously kept herself alone with me:

Th: When I mentioned that you withdraw from your boyfriend when you're angry, you felt I was attacking you and believed I would disapprove of your need for time alone.

Ct: That is exactly what you were doing (*said with disdain*).

Th: When you said you'd left town for a few days because you needed to get away from him after a disagreement, it sounded like withdrawing. It didn't seem like you were going away on a retreat but rather that your anger led to your pulling away. I could be wrong and I'm sorry to wound you. I know how much you want a relationship to work and I wondered if going away served you?

Ct: Ok. I can see that. (*Undoing a projection onto me that I disapproved of her.*) I suppose this doesn't help anything.

Th: I'm glad this makes sense for you. I do find myself in a quandary sometimes, because you want me to help you to sustain a relationship. If I draw attention to something that could be getting in your way, I can appear critical. This seems like a dilemma.

Ct: I guess I distance pretty rapidly without being aware of it. I just don't trust people. I was hurt when he had a different idea of how to handle our living arrangement.

Th: It seems that your mind made assumptions that he doesn't care about you and that I'm critical of you. It's so sad that you'll cut yourself off from a process in which you can talk about your needs and his and find a way through these conflicts. (*She told me later that this exchange had an empowering effect on her.*)

Exposing Latent Yearnings

I received a beautiful note of appreciation from a client, a therapist who ventured into artistic pursuits. I told her I would never discard her card because it touched me profoundly, and I believed she had a remarkable gift for writing. She started tentatively:

Ct: I wouldn't want to make a resolution (*She stopped her sentence abruptly. Frequently, comments that begin with "I don't want" or "I don't feel" camouflage an opposite desire. I almost feel sorry for the defensive system when negation reveals the true story. My client's halting words invited me to dismiss them, but we need to tune in to what the client ignores.)*

Th: A resolution to ...? (*She thought about her upcoming retirement*)

Ct: I want to devote this next phase of my life to *new* forms of creative expression. I plan to write. (*Her voice lowered, making it hard to hear her. I saw her vulnerability as she unmasked her dream. I felt in my gut that something was being born. Suddenly we both erupted in a happy celebration as one of her original therapeutic goals had been to find artistic expression in a new medium.*)

Without a Destination, How Do We Know When We Arrive?

Aimlessness operating in treatment rarely feels useful to either partner. Yet, drifting to nowhere avoids the anxiety of moving somewhere. Therapists sometimes find it tough to raise questions about goals and progress because painful realizations may follow. Maybe the therapy isn't going as well as we'd hoped, or maybe a client has to face the fact that a goal is unattainable. But the truth will win in the end. Better to face reality now than to fail to see problems coming. Doing periodic, honest assessments reenergizes and refocuses therapy.

Toxic Hope

The concept of toxic hope is a revelation for many clients, who suddenly realize they've pursued something for years that isn't possible or would be a disaster. Not all desires deserve the same weight. Some hopes are profound, such as wanting to become a better caretaker to a terminally ill parent and wanting to overcome feelings of resentment about the sacrifice involved. This aspiration benefits both the client and the loved one, which is true of many healthy desires. Some desires ensure failure and disappointment because they're superficial, ill-advised, or impossible. For example, "I'd like you to help me to become more motivated to exercise a minimum of five hours daily because that helps me to look my best. This routine would solve my problems." Maybe someone asks the therapist to help them leave a spouse. A man may perceive that his wife feels disgust toward him, but he has projected his belief that he is repugnant onto her. As a result, he may not absorb her loving feelings for him. What if he bases his wish to divorce on toxic projections? I might say:

> *Th:* I hear your desire to escape your marriage. Yet, depression and feelings of worthlessness have been with you for years, long before you met your wife. Your depression will impact how you view your marriage and yourself. What if we were to work to lift your depression before you make such a big decision?

A female client said she wants to fix what's wrong with her because her husband had another affair, something he had done with his previous two wives. The client believes if she could perfect herself, he will become faithful. Toxic hope causes agony when people work toward changing another person who doesn't want to change. I want to help my client see this truth and also to protect our relationship by reducing false expectations. I had to talk to her about her desire that reality be other than it is. Three women had been unable to change her husband's behavior. Why would she have this power now? Would she want to look at why she assumes that she is deficient? We'd be more likely to see results with such a goal.

> *In another illustration, a young man consulted me about his marital difficulties. He said he had good relationships except with his wife, who had a pattern of verbally abusing him.*

> *Ct:* I want to be more attentive to my wife and be the man she wants.

> *Th:* I see that you've worked hard to please your wife. You also said that your wife was depressed and dissatisfied for years before you met her. You suggested several couple's therapists, and she declined. What does this imply to you about your chances of "becoming the man she wants?"

> *Ct:* It doesn't look real hopeful.

> *Th:* Sadly, that seems true. When we hope for something that isn't possible, it's toxic hope because it's so poisonous and destined for failure.

> *Ct:* Toxic hope? I never heard that term before. It feels right. But maybe there's a way?

Th: Do you have any evidence that the future is likely to be different from the past? (*He says no.*) Perhaps we could help you more by exploring your feelings toward your wife if you were to face the futility of changing her?

Just as a therapist can't heal without a joining of wills, so too our clients can't make a relationship work if their partner doesn't collaborate. I could not agree to work with this client toward a goal I didn't believe we could achieve. He can enhance his relationship skills, but molding himself into the man his wife fantasizes goes beyond the scope of psychotherapy. If he wanted to work on self-care and pursue his personal goals, we would have a realistic destination. We need to trust our instincts about what is possible. Truth is of little use if we don't acknowledge it.

Change Starts from within: An Internal Focus

"Implicit hope practices addressed two key aspects of therapy (a) attending to the therapeutic relationship, and (b) fostering client perspective change" (Larsen & Stege, 2010). Being honest about our abilities and limitations builds trust in the therapeutic relationship. As we identify what we cannot control, we simultaneously explore options more likely to succeed, such as shifting from an external to an internal focus. Some examples:

Ct: I want my family to show me more respect (*external focus*).

Th: I've noticed that sometimes you talk over your valuable feelings. If we give more importance to your emotions, others may value your feelings more. I've seen this happen numerous times. How does this idea appeal to you?

Or:

Ct: My boss yells at me.

Th: How awful for you! So how would you hope we can help you to deal with this terrible reality? Your boss may continue to yell. What would you hope might be different inside yourself? (*The client might identify a desire to reduce anxiety, depression, become more assertive, or find the courage to change jobs. All would shift the work to an internal focus.*)

"Patients who were prepared to have realistic expectations of therapy had a better outcome than did controls who received the identical treatment but without preparation" (Hoehn-Saric et al., 1964). Since realistic goals always involve an internal focus, we ask questions like:

> "What are you experiencing inside that you would like us to help you with?"
>
> "What are you hoping would feel different within yourself as a result of our work together? What would success feel like?"

Resist Assumptions about Goals

Jason's therapist referred him to me because she'd been unable to make emotional contact with him after a year of work. He was depressed and had convinced himself he couldn't feel. His wife had left him a couple of years earlier, and he'd gained 70 pounds since then. He was a successful artistic director, but his company laid him off, and he felt unworthy in every area of his life. Also, he'd estranged himself from his father for many months. He felt hopeless. In the first session, I focused on his desires for treatment. He had difficulty stating what he wanted (Warshow, 2010).

Th: Tell me about what you're hoping for in therapy?

Ct: I have no interest in doing things that I used to enjoy (*he clenches and unclenches his fist*). Generally, I spend my time in my apartment on the couch or in the chair, watching TV, or doing some work. (*He hooks his right arm behind his head and sighs, looking detached. He described his habits, but his desires remain unclear.*)

Th: Are you saying that you're missing something? I wondered what you're hoping for in our work together?

Ct: I don't know (*smiles slyly*). What would I be missing? I don't know.

His vagueness around his desires invites me to figure out what he needs. If I go down that road, I implicitly express a lack of faith in him. He came to me for something. If I imposed a sense of direction, he would resist me or become compliant. Neither helps. I wonder, "What motivates him?" He doesn't know what matters to him, or that he matters at all.

Th: Would you want to explore what matters to you, Jason?

Ct: It bothers me that I have to convince myself to go out and do things that should be fun that should be natural. The guys call me and invite me to a hockey game, and I hem and haw over it. On the day of the event, I spent an hour and a half wondering (*smiling nervously*), "Shall I try and get out of this thing?"

Th: Sounds like the struggle to make decisions and socializing torments you.

Ct: (*He nods and bites lip.*) Yeah. The indecisiveness. (*Here, Jason identifies meaningful goals. He wants to be decisive and more comfortable socializing.*)

Th: Would you want us to help you to become more decisive and have less anxiety about socializing? (*Helping him to declare his authentic goals.*)

Ct: Yes. That would be a good thing. (*He identifies two meaningful goals.*)

Th: Great! I'm delighted you helped us clarify what you hope for in our work. Let's make a point to remember these goals as we work together. (*Highlighting the importance of his desires.*)

Making Meaning of Body Signals

The lip-biting is probably a co-mingling of feelings, shame and anxiety, so I ask with tenderness:

Th: Jason, I wonder if it's difficult to tell me about your desires and needs, causing you to suffer from anxiety or shame? (*Social anxiety will be likely in our relationship. The choice of the word "suffer" conveys compassion.*)

Ct: Yeah, I've constantly got muscle tension everywhere in my body, but primarily in my legs, my feet, and sometimes my jaw.

Th: Thanks for telling me what's going on in your body. Even though muscle tension feels very uncomfortable, it tells us your feelings are rising to the surface, and that's good (*he expresses relief*). I'm also sad that something binds your feelings so tightly inside you (*my sadness allows him to feel his own*).

Ct: Yeah. It's making me feel sad, just saying it (*his eyes reveal pain*).

Th: I can see that, and I'm so glad we can both feel this caring for you. I'd like to encourage you to stay here, with this sadness, if that's ok?

Ct: No. I think that's why I'm here (*He sighs, smiles nervously, and bites his lip. It would be easy to overlook that he said, "No," a refusal to stay with his sadness. I respond with softness in my voice.*)

Th: When you say "no" to staying with your sadness, I believe self-protection is operating, which will sadly perpetuate your suffering—your indecision, your avoidance of hanging out with your friends, and even your weight gain. These signs of depression grow from a need to shut down unbearable pain and withdraw. But isolating is the root source of most emotional pain. (*He nods in agreement.*) Something in you wants you to detach, shut down, "veg out," and withdraw from life (*he nods in agreement again*), causing you to avoid things that could be fun and enriching. Fear and possibly shame of your emotional self-cuts you off from others. (*He reflects a few moments and nods once more.*)

Th: Does this make sense for you?

Ct: Sure. I guess when I say "no" to that question, it's not a conscious "no." Consciously, I understand that there's a need for me to deal with this crap. Otherwise, I wouldn't be here. It gets to a point where it comes up to about here (*pointing his right hand to a place just below his throat*), and then it chokes me (*fighting tears*).

Th: Yes, something chokes off your tears while another part of you wants you to be free to feel and connect. I hear that you wish to stay with the sadness (*highlighting his desire to feel*).

Ct: Yes, absolutely. (*He nods emphatically.*)

Th: You do feel the willingness? (*Reaffirming his will to feel.*)

Ct: Yes. (*With his declaration of will, I return to an exploration of his feelings.*)

Th: That's good! Tell me, what do you notice inside your body as you feel the sadness?

Ct: (*Looking downward) I feel ashamed and unworthy to have a date, to be accepted by a woman.* (*Since I am a woman, I believed he was telegraphing that I won't accept him either. I explored this probable projection directly.*)

Th: You don't know me, and it takes courage to open up to a stranger. I sense you're working hard to be authentic with me, and I appreciate that effort. It makes me sad that you see yourself as so undesirable and I wonder what you experience with me? (*Bringing his attention to our relationship.*)

Ct: You seem to care. I feel like my hand has become really light (*his brow furrows, and he chews his lip as he fights back tears*). I don't feel sad right now (*his mouth trembles, barely noticeable, as he denies his sadness*).

Th: Let me first say that you're right. I do care. But as we attempt to draw closer, I sense that you become anxious and ashamed because you don't expect me to care. Feelings rise, and fear causes lightness in your hands, muscle tightness, and it pushes back your tears. (*He nods comprehendingly.*)

Ct: But I don't feel sadness right now. (*He continues to deny that he has feelings.*)

Th: Did you detach? (*Implying that he can choose otherwise.*)

Ct: (*He scratches his left cheek and scrunches his face.*) I think so. I'm feeling something here (*makes a circular motion around his chest area*), but I don't feel sad.

Th: Great that you're aware. What do you notice in your chest?

Ct: Some anxiousness.

Th: What do you imagine this anxiety is about, with me now?

Ct: Well, I just met you (*smiling shyly*).

Th: Of course. It's natural to feel anxious, meeting me for the first time (*normalizing his anxiety*). Yet, despite your fears, you let us know about the tightening in your throat every time your tears want to surface. I wonder if there's something about my seeing your tears that makes this hard too (*directly addressing shame*)?

Ct: Or letting anybody see my sadness. It's not something I want to do. It just doesn't feel right. (*I'm imagining others have shamed him for showing his emotions in the past.*)

Th: You have every right not to share your feelings, and you don't have to do anything for me. I'm here to help you, and I have no expectations of you (*reducing the pressure to please me*). I imagine you don't yet feel safe with me or perhaps with anyone? Sadly, others have damaged your trust. However, your distrust stands in the way of your freedom to get together with your friends and to date. You believe that you're unworthy and question why anyone would want to be with you. How do you imagine I'm feeling toward you? (*Addressing shame and exploring his projections onto me.*)

Recalling and restating the client's desires in his own words shows that his goals have meaning to me. Hope awakens in him as I spoke to the part that desires something better for himself and expressed compassion for his conflict. He has over-identified with his depressed, unworthy self, and I wanted to draw attention to his wise, observing self who seeks a better future. As his will comes online, a significant shift in gears occurs as his unguarded and truest desires emerge.

Ct: Hmm, you brought up something interesting. It seems like the only person I've ever shown my emotions to is my son. (*His lips quiver, and he averts my eyes as he chokes impulses to cry.*)

Th: You feel the safest with him, and he means the world to you.

Ct: Yeah (*sighing*). It tears me up that I've hurt him, that I've disappointed him. (*He wells up with tears of guilt and pain.*)

Th: Just let it come. That's how I can help you the most. Just let it come.

This last exchange was pivotal. Jason's grief and guilt broke through. A fierce desire to provide his son with a more intimate relationship than he'd had with his dad became a driving force in his treatment. The strength of his newfound purpose had power beyond anything he and I could have engineered. When his unconscious yearnings took the lead, doors opened, and he shared a memory that popped into his mind. He'd been fly fishing and saw a dad and son on the opposite bank of the river. The father was loudly scolding his son. Jason identified deeply with the boy, and this recollection unleashed violent rage impulses toward his father. His river of feelings began to flow. After he destroyed his father in a fantasy for having humiliated him many times, grief and love broke through, which led to a desire to reconnect with his dad. At the end of our first three hours, we had this exchange:

Th: It strikes me how far you've come. What a huge step for you to let me in, a stranger! You know, you are in a very different place from where we began. (*He nods in agreement, smiling.*)

Ct: Yeah, I know that. It felt natural.

Th: How does that feel to make room for this kind of intimacy with someone you just met and feel natural about it?

Ct: It feels kind of weird (*smiles shyly and chuckles*). It's just—it's different. It's different. I always felt like I was so socially inept (*smiling*

> *shyly*), and to think that I can sit down here and talk to you about the deepest, darkest things. It should be a learning experience to me that I can talk to pretty much anybody about anything.

This declaration suggested the birth of new circuitry in the brain. He no longer linked emotional transparency with shame, ridicule, and loss. Jason's relationship with me and himself is different from anything he'd known before. When healing attachment experiences repeat themselves, both inside and outside the office, we can expect change. He later resumed his relationship with his father on terms that would not be detrimental to him. He spent more time with his friends and broke free of his depression. In my last contact with him, he had started to date.

When dormant needs or desires awaken, they give birth to a "visceral vision" for oneself that brings forth healing. Such a vision must be called into existence through mutual caring. Our clients feel these longings in the body before words form, and these desires are often first expressed through tears. I am moved by the client's newfound freedom to declare his desires and feelings with me. Liberation often stirs grief in the client for what was lost and now is found.

References

Berg, I. K., & Dolan, Y. (2001). *Tales of solutions: A collection of hope-inspiring stories*. W. W. Norton & Co.

Bresler, J., & Starr, K. (Eds.). (2015). *Relational psychoanalysis and psychotherapy integration: An evolving synergy*. Routledge/Taylor & Francis Group.

Frank, J. D., & Frank, J. B. (1993). *Persuasion and healing: A comparative study of psychotherapy*. Johns Hopkins University Press.

Hoehn-Saric, R., Frank, J. D., Imber, S. D., Nash, E. H., Stone, A. R., & Battle, C. C. (1964). Systematic preparation of patients for psychotherapy: Effects on therapy behavior and outcome. *Journal of Psychiatric Research*, *2*(4), 267–281. https://doi.org/10.1016/0022-3956(64)90013-5

Horvath, A. O., & Greenberg, L. S. (Eds.). (1994). *The working alliance: Theory, research, and practice*. Wiley & Sons.

Ilardi, S. S., & Craighead, W. E. (1994). The role of nonspecific factors in cognitive-behavior therapy for depression. *Clinical Psychology: Science and Practice*, *1*(2), 138–156. https://doi.org/10.1111/j.1468-2850.1994.tb00016.x

Imber, S. D., Pande, S. K., Frank, J. D., Hoehn-Saric, R., Stone, A. R., & Wargo, D. G. (1970). Time-focused role induction. *Journal of Nervous and Mental Disease, 150*(1), 27–30. https://doi.org/10.1097/00005053-197001000-00004

Koestler, A. (1964). *The act of creation.* Macmillan.

Larsen, D. J., & Stege, R. (2010). Hope-focused practices during early psychotherapy sessions: Part 1: Implicit approaches. *Journal of Psychotherapy Integration, 20*(3), 271–292. https://doi.org/10.1037/a0020820

Luborsky, L. (1976). Helping alliances in psychotherapy. In J. L. Clegh- horn (Ed.), *Successful psychotherapy* (pp. 92–116). Brunner/Mazel.

Warshow, S. (2010). The impact of desire and hope in defeating resistance. *AD HOC Bulletin of Short-Term Dynamic Psychotherapy, 6*(1).

Wickramasekera, I. (1985). A conditioned response model of placebo effect: Predictors from the model. In L. White, B. Tursky & G. Schwartz (Eds.), *Placebos: Theory, research, and mechanisms* (pp. 255–287). Guilford Press.

Wilkins, W. (1979). Expectancies in therapy research: Discriminating among heterogeneous nonspecifics. *Journal of Consulting and Clinical Psychology, 47*, 837–845. https://doi.org/10.1037/0022-006X.47.5.837

Wilkins, W. (1985). Placebo controls and concepts in chemotherapy and psychotherapy research. In L. While, B. Tursky & G. Schwartz (Eds.), *Placebos: Theory, research, and mechanisms* (pp. 83–109). Guilford Press.

4

FORGING A LIFE-ALTERING ALLIANCE

What is a robust working alliance in psychotherapy? Both partners join forces toward specific goals, with a mutual understanding of the process to achieve the desired results. Paradoxically, by agreeing on a framework, we create spaciousness for unlimited, meaningful exploration. An authentic therapeutic relationship requires fluidity and flexibility guided by principles and a dedication to relieve suffering. Throughout every phase of the therapeutic process, the therapist seeks to establish a genuine connection. Sometimes, this involves an occasional detour to share something in common (e.g., a passion for basketball) or laugh together at something silly. Every moment does not have to be "on task" The therapist tries to decipher between significant distractions to avoid feelings or an occasional detour that forges a bond. Most importantly, the therapist attempts to sustain a focus on the path to the most profound material.

The framework generates hope and safety while creating a partnership. As clients clarify their aims for treatment, they wonder, "So how do we get there?" "What is the role of each partner?" "How do we know when we're moving forward or treading water?" Clarity about the process of therapy lays the foundation for a better outcome. In reality,

DOI: 10.4324/9780429399633-5

therapy partners become fuzzy about their roles in the change process. When we run into resistance, the therapist may begin to overwork, and the client may become less involved as a result.

The following exchange involves a client who moved beyond her chronic depression in therapy. We'd had a strong therapeutic alliance but hit a road bump after she returned from a vacation. She had risked being more transparent with her family, but they resisted the changes in her. When we started the session, she began to shut down. I resisted overworking so she could clarify her struggles and choices:

Ct: I'm tired, and I don't want to be here. I'd rather be napping. But I'm here. I had my commitment, so I kept it.

Th: A commitment to—?

Ct: Myself.

Th: So there's a part of you that doesn't want to show up for yourself? It wants to check out.

Ct: That's what I want to do. Check out. None of it makes a difference.

Th: This is a change from where you were last session. You came in saying you felt so good. You were perceiving something shifting. And then somewhere along the way...

Ct: Yeah, I fall back into the same patterns. It's a comfortable shoe. It's a lot of effort to change. It's upsetting the apple cart with everybody around. It's just easier to retreat and keep the status quo.

Th: And end up not living, which is why you came here?

Ct: Right.

Th: So there's a high cost. (*Remembering the cost of the defenses can't be overemphasized.*)

Ct: Yeah. I agree with you. There is a big cost.

Th: There's a cost either way.

Ct: Yeah, so it's like, which is more costly?

Th: Yes. You have conflicting voices. There's a voice that tells you to retreat and maintain the status quo. There's another part that doesn't want you to stop your efforts to find fulfillment in your life, which is the part that comes in here today. Do you want to give voice to the part that comes to see me today?

Ct: The part that shows up says, "This is worthwhile," but the other part says, "To what end?"

Th: What's the payoff for showing up?

Ct: I'll get out of this depression and have a life. (*It's far more potent to allow the client to find answers.*)

Later in the session:

Th: I think of myself as a Sherpa, taking people up the mountain of their choosing. I'm familiar with the route. I'd love for you to reach the peak, but I wouldn't try to pull you up there against your will. That would disrespect you. It's a climb for both of us, and I won't attempt it without you choosing to join me. Does this make sense for you?

Ct: Yeah. It has to be a partnership.

Th: Exactly. Can you imagine a Sherpa taking somebody up Everest if a significant part of that person does not want to go or feels it's better to stay at—

Ct: —basecamp. (*I love when clients join me in the creation of metaphors.*)

Th: Right. I think that's where we are.

Ct: I haven't even gotten to the first camp?

Th: I think you did, and then you said, "That's high enough, I don't want to climb anymore." And the old patterns dominated you.

Ct: Yes.

Th: Now, what do we do? (This question helps clarify our next step, sustaining momentum.)

Ct: I think we trudge forward one foot at a time up the hill. I think it's ultimately better for me, even if it doesn't feel like it is. (*She owns her own decision.*)

Th: Do you remember what you felt before when you were climbing with me?

Ct: It felt very good.

Division of Responsibilities

Let's take a look at what the therapeutic climb means for both partners. What is the therapist's role and the client's role if the trek is to succeed? Therapists take on a huge burden when they forget this division of responsibility. We do not assign responsibility to our clients, as they are not required to do anything. However, both partners need to engage in the process to get the mutually desired results.

A **The therapist's role:**

1 **Invite the client to reveal desires for therapy** (including descriptions of internal suffering and hopes for change)

a **Explore multiple goals**

b **Explore feelings only after the client's goals come into focus** Without goals, there is no reason to explore anything. Avoid making assumptions about what the client wants or hurrying. Re-clarify the client's objectives throughout treatment. "We are helping the dreamer acknowledge and preserve a cherished hope and belief" (Borenstein, 2003).

2 **Recommend a partnership involving mutual, caring attention to feelings, bodily sensations, thoughts, and reflections on the therapeutic relationship occurring in the present moment** Explicitly state that the therapist has no expectations and will honor the client's choices (not always easy to do). One client said to me, "I want stress reduction techniques only." I knew I was not a good fit for this client and suggested a referral.

Thoughts may include beliefs related to religious or spiritual experiences. When the client initiates these topics, we explore these beliefs for their psychological impact, either positive or negative.

3 **If the client chooses this partnership, begin to explore for feelings related to the presenting problem involving feelings toward the therapist, a current or past figure**

4 **Employ the "Healing Triad" (next chapter) when the barriers of toxic shame, anxiety, guilt, and self-protective strategies (SAGSS) appear**

Help the client to identify these obstacles and distinguish the self-enhancing from the self-hurting parts within themselves. Bring the costs of SAGSS to awareness and express verbal and embodied compassion for the suffering they cause. We hope the therapist's compassion will transfer to the client (the "Therapeutic Transfer of Compassion for Self"). Often, the TTCS leads to the "Mobilization of the Will" to embrace feelings and form an intimate human connection.

5 **Shift gears to begin a full exploration of feelings once we've regulated the barriers to emotional connection (SAGSS)**
This involves inquiry into feelings, tracking bodily sensations to see if there is activation associated with core feelings, and using imagery to envision the release of the impulses. It's most important to work with any barriers to complex feelings at this stage, which may include rage, grief, and love.

6 **Guide the client toward co-creating meaning from a session or the therapy overall.**
This step is collaborative. Together, recall the client's goals and presenting problems. Review the barriers to feelings that the client overcame. Acknowledge the feelings and repressed memories that emerged. Reflect on the meaning and purpose of these feelings and memories. Explore how the client can integrate and apply them to the client's current life. Explore how the past was experienced as a child and consider the new narrative that has evolved through treatment.

B **The client's role:**
With the therapist's support and guidance, the client hopefully develops enough self-caring and will to enact the following:

1 **I choose to explore and identify my personal goals**

2 **I choose to observe and share my internal process** (feelings, bodily sensations, thoughts)

3 **I choose to identify and release toxic forms of SAGSS** (shame, anxiety, guilt and self-protective strategies) that inflict incalculable suffering

4 **I choose to access my feelings**
I discover that my will can overcome barriers to feelings and allow my true feelings to emerge.

5 **I choose to share repressed memories that rise to awareness**
I join my therapist to make meaning from my life experiences. I discover the origins of my defensive processes and recognize how each of the SAGSS has poisoned my life. What operations within myself do I want to leave behind? Conversely, what aspects of myself do I want to magnify as I enter the outside world?

6 **I intend to exercise my newfound freedom to enjoy secure relationships based on mutual authenticity**

Tracking the Partnership

A new client, Jackie, was sharp and successful. She exposed her vulnerability saying she was terrified she couldn't sustain a relationship. I wondered what would need to shift inside her to turn this tragic situation around? As she told me about her disappointments in relationships and her prior therapies, I caught a flash of shame in her eyes, which receded rapidly. But my body registered a tiny jolt, which I didn't want to ignore. Our exchange went like this:

Ct: I've had quite a few relationships, and I don't know if my current one will make it. My therapies haven't worked out so well, either. (*She was referred by her couple's therapist, who confirmed that her relationship is in crisis.*)

Th: Are you in therapy now?

Ct: I've decided to stop. I haven't been able to make use of my therapy, and we spent a lot of time on things that felt irrelevant to me. You came highly recommended, but I don't have much hope. I've been at this for years.

Th: I felt something happen inside me as you were speaking (*a mini-electrical current*). Is it ok with you if we pause and talk about how it is for you to share yourself with me?

Ct: It's depressing. I feel very exposed.

Th: Yes. Something told me that these experiences are difficult to talk about and that you're drawing on courage. I feel empathy for you. (*We sit in silence.*)

Ct: I may be so damaged that I may be unable to make use of any therapy. (*She looks down.*)

Her intimate disclosure tells us she doubts that either of us can help her, a belief that could crush every effort we make together. The next exchange about her shame sets the stage for forging a potentially meaningful partnership.

Th: How do you imagine I'm reacting to your doubts that we can succeed together?

Ct: You won't want to work with me.

Th: I'm genuinely touched you would share this. Again, your courage impresses me. Might you be describing how you see yourself, judging yourself as hopeless and unworthy of our efforts? Your view of your deficiencies gives you the impression that I see you in the same way, but do we have any confirmation this is true?

Ct: I know this comes from me (*recognizing her projection onto me*). You're not showing any signs of not wanting to work with me.

Th: In fact, I feel encouraged by your brave leap of intimacy. You're letting us know that some part of you tells you that you're hopeless, and no one would want you. Would you want us to give special attention to this shaming voice that views both of us as inadequate to help you or to care for you? It seems like this voice could convince both of us to give up. Could we look at this part of you without judgment as it informs us where you are hurting?

Ct: I've never considered this before. What you're saying gives me hope.

Her facial muscles relax in relief. Her shoulders drop as she considers an alternative to being at the mercy of forces that devalue both of us. (She and her feelings of shame are not merged. Undoing her shame emerges as a purpose for our work.)

Th: I'm so glad. I experience you as being authentic with me, even though it's difficult to reveal yourself (*she nods*). Your realness bodes well for your therapy. You've shown your sadness and pain, your shame, and a sense of hopelessness. (*Reinforcing her ability to participate meaningfully in our partnership.*) I encourage you to continue noticing all that arises within you—feelings, thoughts, and body sensations, with as little judgment as possible.

Ct: I'm afraid I can't keep it up, and I'll forget.

Th: I promise you that I will forget things too, Jackie, but can't we help each other out when either of us overlooks something important? (*She smiles broadly with relief, perhaps because she senses that she has an ally and it's ok for both of us to have limitations.*) It would also help us to notice any shifts in our relationship as it progresses.

Ct: I like the sound of this approach, but I'm not good at it, seeing what I'm experiencing.

Th: No one is good at this without practice. Would you want me to guide you?

Ct: I think that's the right way to go. (*I've explicitly described my suggested path to help her—confidently because I believe in it—and she has become conscious of how she can help us succeed.*)

Th: Tell me about your most recent relationship with your therapist.

Ct: She seemed to have an agenda. Some of it was useful, but she'd talk a lot about her ideas that I found to be a waste of my time.

Another client told me once that she'd felt tortured for ten years by her analyst's remoteness. Whether she perceived this accurately or not, it serves for the therapist to check out the state of the relationship often. "How do you feel about this exchange between us?" "How do you hear my words?" "How do you feel about the direction we're taking?" "It looked like a feeling crossed your face. Could we see what you're feeling about me?" We then need to give our clients the space to reflect. We can easily make assumptions about how the client responds to us that may be far from reality.

Th: Where did your feelings go when your therapist shared thoughts that felt irrelevant to you?

Ct: I try to be a "good girl," and eventually, I'm out the door.

Th: So, being a good girl (*complying*) leads to your relationships ending? This statement is significant. Your feelings become suppressed as you try to be pleasing, and then you ultimately withdraw. Then you feel like you've failed and that you're alone. You just made a vital link. You've identified that putting your feelings aside and driving them outside your consciousness guarantees that your relationships will fall apart. Does that sound right to you?

Ct: I'm on the verge of leaving my partner now, and I've left quite a few. You're right. I withdraw and believe there's no point in expressing myself.

Th: Tragically, you came to believe that your feelings will have no impact on others, that you will be abandoned, and that you're incapable of caring for yourself. A cruel shaming force has taken root inside of you.

Ct: I hadn't thought of it as shame before. But you're right. I don't feel like I deserve anything.

Th: Someone taught you to feel this way. I believe your discouragement underestimates both of us. What if the relationship you need most begins inside of you—caring for yourself in a way that values your feelings and your needs? Is this something you'd want for yourself? (*As I treated her emotions like they mattered, she began to cry, and anxiety rose.*) Tell me what you're feeling now.

Ct: Yes. I know you're right (*wiping away tears*). I'm not going to find what I'm looking for entirely from the outside. But I'm fearful. I don't know how this will come to be.

Th: I have faith that the two of us could overcome this shaming force inside you by gently drawing our awareness to your internal experience—noticing when your shame is doing a number on you and seeing if we can't move past it—so we can give attention to your feelings and other signals within your body. Is this something you'd want to try with my help?

Ct: Yes. I have to try. I have no other option.

Her pattern of withdrawing when complex feelings are activated will undoubtedly occur in our relationship too. If we're not paying attention to her shame and her distancing defenses, her feelings will become submerged, and she'll drop out of therapy. Her new awareness—that shame causes her to pull away from everyone she gets close to, including herself, and costs her dearly—will hold value if she cares sufficiently for herself to forge a life-altering partnership with me.

We will work together to give caring attention to her feelings, bodily sensations, beliefs, and the state of our relationship. This process is similar to a meditative practice that allows phenomena within us to rise to awareness with acceptance.

Two primary elements of a change-oriented alliance emerged

1 We clarified the client's goals
   A The ability to sustain a long-term relationship
   B Freedom from crippling shame
   C Expression of feelings rather than withdrawal from them
   D Attention to her internal experience

2 We agreed on a path to help her sustain a relationship

Client Permission

Our clients may not accept our suggested path. Out of respect, we honor their choices, making space for them to differentiate from us. The approach we prefer may not be theirs. Our willingness to let go of the outcome makes us better therapists, even though this increases our sense of risk. It's a price worth paying. Often the client is unaware of what the therapist is doing or why. The client wonders: "Why is the therapist asking me these questions?" "Where is the therapist heading?" "What does the therapist expect of me?"

A therapist may inquire into a client's bodily sensations without recognizing that these questions can feel invasive. The fact that someone seeks therapy doesn't mean they've granted permission to enter their private world. We can achieve positive results without an explicit agreement, but then we may fail to build selfhood. We're proceeding without collaboration, and in my opinion, the ends do not justify the means. A *shame sensitive* approach seeks conscious permission to embark upon a chosen path, which telegraphs faith in the client's wisdom and healing capacity. Some examples:

> "Would it be ok with you if we give attention to your bodily sensations since our bodies provide such invaluable information about what we're feeling?"
>
> "It's been my experience that attention to your feelings reduces anxiety. However, I want to honor your choices, and I'm interested in your reaction to the idea of focusing on your feelings?"

While seeking the client's consent periodically takes more time and effort, respect for autonomy pays off. Research suggests that a collaborative process is healing (Tryon et al., 2018). By definition, the "other" is different from "me," and regardless of my fantasies, skills, and intuition, I cannot know the other if I fail to inquire. Even if my responses have merit, it means nothing if the client has no use for them. Undigested food provides no nourishment. When the client agrees with my recommended approach compliantly but veers away from an internal focus in reality, the alliance is inactive.

A supervisee presented such a case to me. The client's unconscious desire to hide was more potent than her will to become aware of her feelings. She pulled the therapist away from a therapeutic focus with various deflections. The therapist asked me to enact a role-play of a typical exchange with her client, where she felt stuck. The following vignette illustrates my suggested responses to her client. As we read the client's statements, let's listen carefully to her internal conflict about drawing attention to herself. I suggested that her therapist bring these dueling parts of herself to awareness, so she would have a chance to move beyond her paralyzing shame states.

The following interactions clarify that the therapist doesn't require the client to give importance to her feelings. Instead, the client chooses to recover a relationship to herself.

Ct: I should be able to begin this conversation (*laughing nervously, sitting sideways, and repositioning her purse repeatedly*). Other people certainly have no problem talking about themselves.

Th: It's good you're noticing that you have difficulty giving attention to yourself, while others have no trouble focusing on themselves. How do you feel when people draw attention to themselves?

Ct: They seem self-centered, full of themselves, and their importance. I know our sessions should be time for me, but I don't even think about our conversations between our meetings (*laughing nervously*). Speaking about self-centered people, George took over the room at a party last week and didn't realize how much talking he does. I could see the look in my girlfriend's eyes when he started giving his opinions.

Th: Would you mind if we pause for a moment, Gretchen, because you said something important? (*Wait to see if she agrees.*) You seem to be saying that you should be able to focus on yourself in your therapy, but your mind also judges others for drawing attention to themselves. You are conflicted about the idea of giving attention to yourself. Tell me about the part of you that believes you should focus on yourself and initiate our conversations?

Ct: I know I have to talk about myself when I see you if I'm going to get anywhere. I just have trouble doing it.

Th: I'm glad you let us know you have trouble initiating our conversations and that when people talk about themselves, it turns you off (*reinforcing her transparency*). I wonder if we could distinguish between people focusing on themselves in ways that exclude others versus you and I making you the center of our attention so you can heal?

Ct: Mmmm. I hadn't looked at it that way.

Th: Yeah. You and I would be making the session about you, so you can receive our attention and care. I noticed a bit of nervous laughter the minute you started to focus on yourself, as if some force silenced you, causing you to feel uncomfortable in your own skin. How sad this seems! How do you feel about what I'm saying?

Ct: Yeah. It is sad. I do feel uncomfortable putting myself out there, being the center of attention. And it bothers me when others get attention, but I feel ashamed when I focus on myself.

Th: When you see others getting attention, you unconsciously yearn for it while judging your desires. What do you sense is causing this self-criticism and shame? How do you imagine I will react if you focus on yourself and your feelings? (*Shame is an interpersonal phenomena related to being seen unfavorably by another. Therefore, I wished to explore any projections onto me, and we discovered a few.*)

Ct: You may find me unattractive, like my ex-husband and my father did. They used my feelings against me. My dad mocked me if I cried. He'd get this disgusted look on his face like I was weak and pathetic. My husband just walks away and seems to do the opposite of what I ask deliberately.

Th: How painful for you! It all makes sense why you'd be silent and keep your feelings hidden (*normalizing her self-protective strategies*). Yet we're in a different time and space now, and you're seeking something new and better for yourself (*reminding her that her trauma is in the past*). Doesn't this devaluing part of you increase your anxiety and deprive you of the attention you deserve from us? (*Submerging her needs also prevents her from pursuing what she wants from her husband and others.*) In truth, as I get to know the real you, I feel closer to you. I like it when you let me know about your needs, your internal struggles, and the discomfort they cause you (*providing a more secure relationship*). How is it to hear me say these things?

Ct: It's really different. I'm starting to feel sad.

The client begins to share her therapist's sadness for her painful trap. As she sees how fear and undeserved shame cause her to hide her needs and deprive her, perhaps she'll want to risk more exposure. The patterns she cannot see will replay endlessly. As I supervise her therapist, I'm struck by the therapist's perceptive, intuitive observations and notice a parallel process. The therapist often pulls back and silences her voice in the session, internalizing what she is experiencing. Both partners lose the benefits of the therapist's observations.

Sometimes our clients mirror our difficulties. I ask the therapist how it would feel to expose her insights and feelings with her client? She realizes she fears taking the lead, interrupting, injecting her point of view, and revealing her feelings. The treatment process stretches both partners simultaneously, and we find that practicing therapy can be therapeutic for us too!

The work of therapy poses a tremendous risk to archaic parts of the self that no longer serve a useful purpose. I once envisioned a graveyard filled with discarded teachings from individuals who loved me or perhaps influenced me through their writings or modeling. Some of these messages were poisonous. However, others held timeless value. The maturation process calls upon us to separate the teachings that serve our mental, emotional, and spiritual evolution from those that do not.

As we sit across from a resistant or fragile client, we both face a challenge. What must each of us release within ourselves to make it possible to form a deeper connection and birth something new? Each of us will have to gently let go of parts of ourselves and tenderly coax other parts into a fuller existence. I remember an experience as a young adult, hiking with a group of friends in the mountains of Northern California. We came upon a ravine. To continue, we had to cross a plank that stretched above a creek bed that lay far below us. One by one, my friends scampered across the piece of wood. When it was my turn, I blithely followed them until I reached the middle of the plank and became aware that if I were to lose my balance and fall, I could break my neck and die.

I desperately wanted to turn around and go back to safety but realized with horror that I would fall if I did. I was in a freeze state. On the other side of the ravine, my friend extended his strong hand and looked at me with steady, penetrating eyes. His wordless look compelled me to walk toward him. I "knew" I had no choice. I had to trust my body and him. This memory brings up fear and gratitude right now. I might not be here were it not for his quick and perfect response. His confidence in me inspired me to make it across. My paralyzing fear and images of breaking my neck had to die for me to live.

Similar fears can beset our clients or us as we venture onto the perceived plank that stretches over a relational abyss. Each of us intensely wants to make it to the other side to experience a secure attachment and a satisfying therapeutic outcome. Gretchen wanted relief from her anxiety and painful aloneness, but she also wanted to avoid her anxiety by returning to her familiar yet costly distancing ways. As therapists, we want to be effective, and we know this requires risk. We also want to hold onto safety. When either the therapist or client feels anxious about trying something new, it's a good sign that we're working on the cusp of change.

In my first session with Karen, we will see how she and I established a partnership that laid a foundation for the risk-taking ahead, allowing her to break free of chronic depression:

Th: I'm happy to meet you. Please tell me what is going on inside you that causes you to seek help?

Ct: Well, a lot of it—I have this consistent feeling when I wake up in the morning, the day is black—kind of like a hollow feeling. And intellectually, I look at my life, and I say there is no reason for this. But it's just how I feel. Every day, it's like, "Okay, today is going to be a good day. You're going to put a smile on your face, and away we go." But there is this kind of nagging undertow. I'm sad. It's a pervasive sadness. People don't know it. I'm very good at hiding it.

Th: It sounds like you're depressed. Tell me more about what you're experiencing?

Ct: I watch TV all day, and I don't want to see my friends. I adore my children, have a long-term marriage, and two beautiful homes. I've done really well in my career. I've been taking antidepressants and don't understand why I feel so hopeless. Maybe because I lost my dad at 18, and my parents were Holocaust survivors. (*Karen saw herself as privileged and believed that "So many have it worse." While this was true, Karen still suffered and deserved care.*)

Th: You've created a full life! But sadly, you're not enjoying it.

Ct: I don't take credit for any of it.

Th: How very sad! I'm curious how you respond to your children's achievements? (*If she can acknowledge others, she can direct a similar appreciation toward herself.*)

Ct: My son just got a great job. I worked for two days to prepare a dinner party for him. I'm very proud of my children.

Th: You celebrate your son's accomplishments with enthusiasm and generosity, but there are no leftovers for you.

Ct: That's why my therapist sent me here. She said, "You need to be as good to yourself as you are to other people." (*She had stopped seeing her therapist ten years ago. Her therapist wanted her to be kinder to herself, but does she want the same? If not, nothing is likely to change. I focus on what she wants for herself, demonstrating that I value her.*)

Th: And how about what you want for yourself? It's excellent you let me know how you're suffering from depression, and I believe you want relief. (*She nods yes.*) But how can you feel happy or motivated without a sense of worth? (*She nods yes.*) Would you want us to see if we can turn this around?

Ct: Yes. I know I don't care much about myself, and I can't go on dragging through each day. It's a very uncomfortable shoe for me (*being kind to herself*), but I don't want to feel crappy.

Th: What brought you to a point where you sought my help? (*Seeking the event that triggered her current depressive episode.*)

Ct: I'm having a hard time coping with my mother because I feel very manipulated by her. And it creates a tremendous amount of anger in me because she expects me to take care of her in a way she never took care of me. I feel guilty for not wanting to help her and also saying no to her.

This amount of insight into her rage and guilt impressed me, yet her awareness alone will not heal her depression. A shame serpent has turned on her, causing her to see herself as fundamentally flawed at her core because of her inability to show tenderness toward her aging, declining mother. I seek to normalize her anger. Compassion is the antidote to shame.

Th: Right. Right. Anyone would have a lot of anger about that. But it wasn't ok for you to feel angry toward your mother. (*I would learn later that her mother subjected her to cruel punishments, locking her outside her home for hours at a time as a young child.*) And so your anger gets submerged and channels into depression (*she agrees*). Fortunately, you're caring for yourself by pursuing therapy again. You show strength by acknowledging your anger, and your guilt tells us that you care about your mother. When your anger can be felt and accepted, it leads to healthy boundaries and the ability to say "No" without guilt. But when anger is not permitted toward your mother, it attacks you by stifling your happiness. It would be great if we could help you experience your feelings without judgment.

Ct: Yeah. That would be a first.

Th: Your awareness is terrific. (*Client laughs dismissively.*) What do you feel when I say that? (*Drawing attention to her self-devaluation is fertile ground.*)

Ct: Umm. Well, there's a part of me that's proud of myself for taking this step and saying, "Enough of the nonsense."

Th: You should be!

Ct: Yeah, well, that's a hard feeling for me (*pride*). It doesn't come naturally. It's uncomfortable.

Mechanisms of suffering defined so far:

1. Depression—likely anger turned on the self, fueled by toxic guilt over rage and submerging complex feelings
2. Unresolved healthy remorse for withholding from her mother
3. Toxic guilt over rage at her mother who cruelly punished her
4. Self-contempt and loathing. Lack of generosity toward herself.

Before exploring Karen's feelings, I want to gain her consent to join me in my approach to psychotherapy. I want to provide full disclosure and reinforce her decision-making power.

Th: I'm very interested in the uncomfortable feelings you're having right now, but I'd like to seek your permission first to explore further. I'd like to share my approach to see if it's ok with you. It matters to me that everything we do is in full partnership with your agreement and understanding. (*Ct: Ok.*) I don't ever want to go someplace you don't want to go. (*Ct: Ok. Ok.*) You've mentioned your history of neglect and putting yourself last in line (*she nods vigorously*). You will care for others and attend to others in ways that you don't show caring for yourself.

Ct: Umm, hmm. Yeah.

Th: I believe that neglect and self-condemnation is fueling your depression. So I suggest that you and I turn this around by giving caring attention to anything you experience internally, such as physical sensations, rising feelings, and beliefs about yourself. It also helps to check how we're doing in our relationship as we sit with each other.

Ct: Ok. (*I need to check for compliance. Does she really agree? What does she feel about my approach?*)

Th: Tell me how you feel about my suggestion?

Ct: It sounds right, but I have no idea how to do it. I'm not good at noticing details.

Th: I'm curious. If I asked you to describe that Kleenex box, could you do it? (*She described the box exactly.*) We see you can recognize details. You're just not used to giving attention to yourself. I'd be with you, guiding you every step of the way. (*Reassuring her she's not alone as she was with her mother, a crucial reminder.*)

Ct: I'm willing to do it, but now I'm feeling very anxious. (*Her anxiety tells us a therapeutic alliance to allow me to know her more intimately is emerging. We began to regulate her anxiety.*)

The alliance that we established in that first session led to wonderful results for her. During treatment, she processed her powerful complex emotions toward her mother and other family members. She became able to care for her mother without resentment while attending to her own needs simultaneously. She no longer felt anxiety around her mother. She was not depressed at the time of termination and was pursuing activities that were deeply gratifying to her.

Many therapists believe that trust and attachment take years to form for the majority of people who seek our help. This idea assumes a time requirement on a person's ability to release toxic processes within themselves and bond in new, healthy ways. If I had believed that healing would take years, much of my work would not have been possible. It's a shame to predetermine the possibilities in human relationships. (Abbass, Town, & Driessen, 2012; Davanloo,1990; Dewan, Steenbarger, & Greenberg, 2017; Fosha, 2000; Greenberg & Safran,1987; Levine, 2008; McCullough Vaillant, 1997; Shapiro, 1995.)

Once my husband and I were lost for hours on side streets in Florence. We might still be going in circles if some kind person hadn't jumped in our back seat and directed us back to our hotel. If we do not show our clients the route to make emotional intimacy and attachment possible, we may be wandering the back roads for a long time. As we forge a therapeutic partnership that makes interpersonal closeness a conscious goal, self-protective responses will challenge us along the way. These mechanisms operate routinely in the client's life, causing damage, so we prefer to bring them into the open sooner rather than later. When we bypass barriers to intimacy, we create a short-lived sense of safety. Isn't it better to show our clients how they can reach the other side of the relationship "plank" by overcoming their fear and dread? Repetitive experiences of relationship safety are the road to secure attachment.

Address Common Obstacles to a Life-Altering Alliance

1 Normalize self-doubts
2 Honor the client's choice in forming an alliance

3 Offer reassurance that the capacity to feel is innate
4 Bring projections into the open to reduce shame
5 Emphasize equality and collaboration to build selfhood
6 Raise awareness of the value of emotions
7 Address a lack of compassion for oneself
8 Acknowledge when the alliance is working or has faltered

Normalize Self-Doubts

When clients consider stepping outside their comfort zones, self-doubts arise. Trying something unfamiliar is poignantly vulnerable and awkward. We feel foolish, silly, stupid, and inept.

Ct: I don't know that I can do this.

Th: Of course. Most people wonder the same thing—will they perform properly and be a "good" client? Is this what it's like for you?

Ct: Yes. I'm afraid of failing.

Th: I empathize with you. All of us have anxiety trying something unfamiliar. But your goals are invaluable, and you will not be alone on this journey. I'm here to guide and support you, and I will not judge you. Tell me honestly if you'd want us to give this work a try?

Honor the Client's Choice in Forming an Alliance

We are suggesting a path, not insisting upon one. The response below has been rare in my practice, but I want to respond respectfully to the client's wishes:

Ct: I'm not sure about your approach. I think I only need some stress-reduction techniques.

Th: Therapists have different approaches to working with stress. I find that giving attention to our emotions can significantly reduce anxiety, and there's quite a bit of research behind that idea. But it's vital that an approach feels right to you.

Ct: I saw some of these techniques on television, and I liked them.

Th: I want to honor your wishes. Therefore, I don't think this approach will be right for you.

Offer Reassurance that the Capacity to Feel is Innate

Clients forget that the ability to experience and share their feelings is innate. If they doubt this reality, invite them to watch children on a playground. Emotions are our birthright, a gift we cannot lose. But feelings need relational encouragement to find appropriate expression:

Th: Our bodies are continually feeling something, but we learn to shut off our awareness of our feelings.

Ct: I'm afraid of the unknown.

Th: That's natural. Everyone is afraid of the unfamiliar. Paradoxically, nothing is more innate and natural than our feelings, yet we can lose touch with them. We could start by noticing that something shuts down your emotions. Would it be ok if we pay attention to anything that pulls you away from what you feel?

We reach feelings by removing the barriers that block them—shame, anxiety, guilt, and self-protective strategies. Feelings will take care of themselves when they feel safe, and we have lifted the barricades to their expression. If it is the client's will to transcend their protective processes, feelings will flow.

Bring Projections into the Open to Reduce Shame

Clients commonly project that the therapist will judge when we explore feelings, and these distortions stifle the uncovering of emotions. We bring projections into the open to deactivate their power. My clients typically assume (project) that I will look at them through their eyes, not mine.

Ct: I'm usually anxious, and it has to do with being a good patient. And doing it right. And doing it...

Th: According to what you imagine I'm expecting.

Ct: Right, right.

Th: Or what you're expecting?

Ct: Yes, according to my standards of being a good patient, being interesting, being in-depth, and bringing something substantial.

Th: So, we see how much you expect of you. Unfortunately, this pressure on yourself squeezes you out of existence. You know, I'm not you. I expect nothing from you, and I'm here only to serve you. I have hopes for you as you do, but hope differs from expectations. (*A comment like this won't stop the projections, but these words reassure.*)

Or:

Ct: My feelings are ugly.

Th: Feelings are neither good nor bad. They just are. When you share what you notice with me, you can make no mistake.

Emphasize Equality and Collaboration to Reduce Shame and Build Selfhood

The therapist holds power as an advisor and expert. A healing relationship is one of equality, shared vulnerability, and mutual respect. Our clients need to impact us as they could not influence their parents. To create a sense of collaboration, we will need the humility to listen and learn from our clients.

Th: You won't be doing this alone. I'll notice what's happening in my body too. Our relationship will benefit when we're both staying connected to ourselves and each other. We'd be doing this as partners. Your feedback will be vital, so I can know if I'm helpful. I won't always be on target, so we'll need to guide each other for the best results. How do you feel about this idea?

Ct: I'll try to be open. It's hard for me.

Th: You're being open now, just telling me this is hard for you! Nothing more nor less is needed. And I'll do my best to be authentic with you. Revealing myself hasn't always been easy for me either. (*Creating equality and shared vulnerability.*)

Raise Awareness of the Value of Emotions

A person is not likely to be motivated to attend to feelings without recognizing the pivotal role of emotions in the quality of life. We can help by raising awareness of the benefits of experiencing emotions: better health; the ability to make intuitive, wise judgments; protection from danger; the motivation to disengage from harmful relationship patterns; an increased capacity for intimacy with others, and a fuller expression of creativity. An illustration of raising awareness of the value of emotions:

Ct: I don't see where feelings are all that useful.

Th: I'm sure you've had experiences that reinforced that belief. Still, you want to make better decisions in your life. How will you be able to do that without a connection to your feelings, as they are your primary compass? You've been operating without access to your feelings for many years. Is it working?

Ct: What I'm doing now needs to change.

Th: Life can't work if we don't know what we feel.

Our clients will discover the value of their feelings once they let themselves feel.

Address a Lack of Compassion for Oneself

The therapeutic alliance won't operate without self-compassion. Attention to our internal experience requires care for ourselves. Is the client willing to direct caring energy toward themselves? Four elements that can activate self-compassion:

A Awareness of the cost of self-protective processes that separate the client from others

B The therapist's compassion for the client's suffering (Have we communicated our caring implicitly and explicitly?)

C A rise of sadness or grief within the client for the losses resulting from defensive processes

D The client's will to direct compassion toward oneself

Example of generating self-compassion:

Ct: I don't like showing my feelings.

Th: You're not sure how much you want to show interest in the silenced parts of yourself?

Ct: I know I need to change, but I don't know how.

Th: If you and I show a caring interest toward your neglected feelings, they will speak to us. Tragically, they've been shoved to the back seat for years (conveying sadness). They cry out for our attention. They must feel wanted and safe to come forward. You show interest when your children are hurt or bullied or disappointed. You would need to shine that same light of caring toward your feelings if you are to experience relief. I'd help you. We would need to inquire, listen, and care. When your feelings are set free, you will have less need to lash out or withdraw, which has cost you relationships. Would you want to try to direct this kind of caring energy toward yourself?

Acknowledge When the Alliance is Working or has Faltered

"The success of all techniques depends on the patient's sense of alliance with an actual or symbolic healer" (Frank & Frank, 1993). Reinforce all forms of transparency to validate the success of the alliance. We can overvalue the breakthrough to feelings and undervalue other forms of intimacy. When a person discloses experiences they've never shared, let's give these moments the appreciation they deserve:

> "It's excellent that you noticed the tightness in your chest and told me that your stomach had seized. Your willingness to share these sensations with me is exactly how we can help you."

> "I'm glad that you shared that you feel suddenly exhausted as we approach your anger. Yet, you have felt energized when you allowed yourself to disclose feelings and be vulnerable. You work tirelessly at your job, but sadly, that same energy dissipates in relation to you. What will be the effect? How do you feel as we notice your fatigue and disengagement from yourself?" (*Clients can swing from barely keeping their eyes open to becoming animated depending on their motivation to engage in the therapeutic process.*)

As therapists, we should feel deeply gratified when we offer a life-altering partnership to our clients who suffer. May we appreciate our efforts as we fulfill our part in the partnership.

References

Abbass, A., Town, J. & Driessen, E.(2012). Intensive short-term dynamic psychotherapy: a systematic review and meta-analysis of outcome research. *Harvard Review of Psychiatry*, 20 (2), 97-108.

Borenstein, L. (2003). The clinician as a dreamcatcher: Holding the dream. *Clinical Social Work Journal*, *31*, 249–262. https://doi.org/10.1023/A:1024080016896

Davanloo, H.(1990). *Unlocking the unconscious: Selected papers of Habib Davanloo*. Wiley.

Dewan, M.J., Steenbarger, B. N., Greenberg, R.P. (2017) (Eds). *The Art and Science of Brief Psychotherapies: A Practitioner's Guide (3rd edition)*. American Psychiatric Publishing.

Fosha, D. (2000). *The transforming power of affect*. Basic Books.

Frank, J. D., & Frank, J. B. (1993). *Persuasion and healing: A comparative study of psychotherapy*. Johns Hopkins University Press.

Greenberg, L.S. & Safran, J.D. (1987). *Emotions in psychotherapy*. Guilford.

Levine, P.A. (2005). *Healing Trauma*. Sounds True.

McCullough Vaillant, L. (1997). *Changing character: Short-term anxietyregulating psychotherapy for regulating, defenses, affects and attachment*. Basic Books.

Shapiro, F. (1995). *Eye movement desensitization and reprocessing: Basic principles, protocols and procedures*. Guilford Press.

Tryon, G. S., Birch, S. E., & Verkuilen, J. (2018). Meta-analyses of the relation of goal consensus and collaboration to psychotherapy outcome. *Psychotherapy*, 55(4), 372–383. https://doi.org/10.1037/pst0000170

5

THE HEALING TRIAD

Bypassing Treatment Barriers

Emotional connection is the lifeblood of relationships and psychotherapeutic healing. When hurdles invariably block the emergence of feelings, the "Healing Triad" provides an orientation to dealing with these challenges with three potent agents of change: 1) raising awareness of treatment barriers (SAGSS, see below) with *shame sensitivity*; 2) the Therapeutic Transfer of Compassion for Self (TTCS); and awakening the will to feel and deeply connect to others. Locking these three elements together in my mind reset my course. First, I discovered that I could not successfully raise awareness of defensive processes without acute attunement to shame. Second, I had to work toward a state of compassion within myself in the face of stubborn treatment barriers. I could then offer my felt compassion as a resource for my client, which I refer to as a therapeutic transfer. Third, I found that this therapeutic transfer of compassion became a primary catalyst in mobilizing the will to feel emotions and increase capacity for secure attachment.

Many authors have richly contributed to the literature on topics directly related to the Healing Triad. (Abbass, 2015; S. Freud, 1894-1958; A. Freud, 1936; Davanloo. 2000; Neborsky, 2001; Frederickson, 2013,

DOI: 10.4324/9780429399633-6

2021; Ecker, 2012; Vaillant, 1997; Fosha, 2000; Alpert, 1992; Coughlin Della Selva, 1996; Neff, 2011, ten Have-de Labije, 2017, and others).

In my effort to raise awareness of barriers, generate self-compassion and mobilize the will, I ran into major stumbling blocks in the quest to achieve emotional intimacy. The Healing Triad incorporates powerful key concepts that allowed doors to closeness to open dramatically with far greater client satisfaction.

The Healing Triad clicked in my mind as I sat wordlessly across from Joanne, who seemed impenetrable. Her thoughts and words bolted and lunged, leaving me trailing behind, and I wasn't sure if she noticed I was in the room. She lived in her head, and her words seemed to go around my ears instead of into them. I wondered, "Is Joanne aware of how anxious she seems and how little attention she pays to her hyperaroused state? Does she know that her rapid, breathless speech prevented us from connecting, overwhelming her and me? Does she notice that she barely sees or hears herself or me?" For Joanne and most of us, our way of being and relating is automatic and unintentional, outside of our awareness.

As I pondered the challenges before Joanne and me, a three-tiered orientation to tackling common obstacles to closeness came together like a tapestry. Now, when I encounter toxic forms of shame, anxiety, guilt, and survival strategies (the SAGSS system), which impedes a fruitful, more profound relationship between my clients and me, I immediately resort to the Healing Triad.

The Healing Triad

1 Raise awareness of Treatment Barriers with *Shame Sensitivity*

The most significant treatment barriers are toxic forms of Shame, Anxiety, Guilt and Self-protective Strategies (SAGSS). These processes can crush well being and derail therapy. SAGSS are in the forefront of my mind as I work always. If you find the acronym hard to remember, think of this:

The human spirit *sags* under the weight of toxic SAGSS!

Each of the SAGSS has healthy and functional forms, but this chapter focuses on the toxic variations that damage the self and relationships:

A Shame—"I am deficient at my core."
B Anxiety—"You will abandon me for showing feelings and desires."

C Guilt—"My feelings harm others, and I deserve punishment."
D Self-Protective Strategies (defenses)—"I need to stay away from you so I won't get hurt or hurt others."

The Healing Triad helped a woman become aware of her shame, anxiety, splitting, and projections. She said the following about her new consciousness:

Ct: I see now. I've been looking at things in a black and white way. (Awareness of splitting.) When I do something, it's never enough. I'm always looking at what I didn't do, not what I did do. (*Th: Right!*) What I left out, what wasn't perfect. So suddenly, there was some kind of switch in my brain, and I looked at myself and started seeing all these perfectionistic ways I'm trying to be in this world, you know? (*The "switch in the brain" telegraphs the organic nature of transformation.*)

Th: Yes!! And in relationships. With me, with others.

Ct: Yes, and in relationships. I've become aware there is anger associated with that. You've helped me see it can come out as a projection. It looks like somebody else is making demands on me. And I do the same by being impatient with my husband when he's not perfect, or being impatient with ...

Th: Or me.

Ct: My kids, or you, expecting something more, but it's usually associated with not feeling good enough inside myself. I started noticing this more from outside myself like, I'm not, I can't explain.

Th: You're doing great!

Ct: It's like, I have a space between me and my anxiety. Before, it was intolerable for me to feel anxious when I was going to do something new. I'd start catastrophizing everything, you know! Immediately it blows up into a disaster inside my brain. Then I started looking at me doing this.

Th: Looking at you terrorizing yourself.

Ct: Yeah. I looked at myself, and it felt ridiculous what I'm doing. It's mind-blowing what I've been doing. How I'm making my life miserable.

Th: It's terrific you have this new awareness of these formerly unconscious forces of anxiety, shame, splitting, and projections that cause you so much suffering! Would you want us to stay aware of these barriers so we can continue to help you to experience the feelings that lie beneath them?

2 Therapeutic Transfer of Compassion for Self (TTCS)

The TTCS begins when the therapist expresses compassion or pain for the trauma that led to the development of SAGSS (toxic Shame, Anxiety, Guilt and Self-protective Strategies) as well as the tragic consequences of these internal saboteurs. The language of compassion is both verbal and embodied. Sometimes the latter carries more impact. When the client is receptive, the therapist's compassion travels between them and takes root in the client. The client awakens to the harm of automatic, lifelong toxic internal processes. What once felt necessary now feels deadly. The therapist's compassion is most likely to impact the client when the therapist expresses:

A Visceral sadness for the severe suffering due to trauma-induced shame, anxiety, guilt and archaic survival strategies (e.g., we show compassion not only for the pain of divorce but for the suffering caused by the emotional numbing that led to the divorce and other fractured relationships)

B Strong advocacy and caring for neglected feelings and desires

C Empathy for tactics of self-camouflage to cope with early injuries, leading to distant relationships and subsequent traumatic losses

D Giving importance to physiological signals that indicate distress in the body and rising emotions

E Compassion that goes beyond verbal expression and includes tender vocal tones, eyes that transmit softness and caring, bodily engagement, and other implicit cues

F A willingness to be emotionally impacted by and to learn from the client

We'll see the TTCS in the following exchange:

Ct: This is so hard to tell you.

Th: I know. I know. (*My voice is tender, and I lean forward with compassion in my eyes.*)

Ct: My mom hit me forcefully for masturbating. (*He looks away with tears streaming down his face.*) I still did it a lot.

Th: It's so natural to find ways to soothe and stimulate yourself, especially when you're terrified and feel so ashamed. (*I place my hand over my heart, feeling pain for him.*) I'm so sad you still feel such shame over your sexuality. Doesn't this shame belong to your mother for attacking you for your natural sexual impulses? (*My voice rises as I advocate for his right to sexual feelings.*) You're so brave to talk to me about this now.

Ct: I never thought about how horribly my mom treated me, only about how bad I was. (He tears up.) You're right. I did nothing wrong and I don't deserve to carry this shame.

3 Mobilization of the Will to Feel and Deeply Connect

When the therapist values the client's feelings and perspectives and the TTCS takes root, the client's will to express emotions often mobilizes.

A Will carries the intention to attend to feelings and desires and also to connect deeply to others. Will is a subtle yet powerful energy force that propels change, occurring both consciously and unconsciously.

B Will arouses the desire to overcome the barriers that block feelings, sabotage one's goals, and prevent nourishing relationships. Will elevates closeness to others to a top priority.

Let's delve further into the Healing Triad's three elements, which will orient us when we encounter most therapeutic challenges.

The Healing Triad—Part I

Awareness of Barriers to Feelings (SAGSS)

Awareness introduces the client to aspects of themselves they hadn't known. A client may say, "I believe this." or "I did that," but we need to ask, what part of oneself initiated this action or belief? Did my eight-year-old self make a decision that impacts me to this day? Would I come to the same conclusion in the present moment? Is there another reality I could access now? Maslow believed that awareness of the self must shift for change to take place.

Many clients are visibly and powerfully impacted when I raise awareness of unconscious patterns that impede relationships, emotional expression, and healthy selfhood. Awareness of SAGSS includes an appreciation for their gritty, resourceful, wise, and amazing aspects. When we address those parts of the self that may have worked in the past but aren't working well today, we want to acknowledge their earlier purpose and value. We might visualize the scales of justice, a symbol of balance, when we work with SAGSS. They represent the person's best efforts to survive the unbearable. When we draw attention to a part of the self that needs to be retired, let's recognize its former usefulness while we highlight those parts that deserve to be born.

Raising awareness of primitive, outdated protective responses that are unconscious will be new for our clients and may surprise, astound, empower, or embarrass them. One man told me he felt a new strength to be able to "track these states like an animal." As he saw how these automatic and reactive threat responses kept him out of a relationship with his wife and two young daughters, he sensed liberation alongside deep regret. When the client felt held in the arms of our co-created compassion, he could courageously look within himself with unwavering honesty. This awakening created profound shifts in his life. Both therapeutic partners promote awareness when they do the following:

1 Name the barriers to closeness (SAGSS—shame, guilt, anxiety, and survival strategies).
2 Notice how SAGSS manifest in the body (e.g., reduced energy, accelerated heart rate, avoidance of eye contact, lip biting, and thought disruption).
3 Identify the tragic costs of SAGSS (e.g., chronic anxiety, depression, avoidance of people, divorce, job loss, isolation, loneliness, and superficial relationships).

These realizations must have an emotional impact, or they remain a distant concept. Always check to see how new awareness lands in the body of the client. "How does it feel inside you to realize that your speech becomes pressured out of anxiety, making it hard for you to connect with people and creating loneliness?"

Another example of raising awareness of SAGSS:

Th: Let me see if I hear you accurately, Carl. You've had a series of disappointments in treatment, and you expect we're likely to fail as well?

Ct: I've tried a lot of different things.

Th: You've had aspirations in therapy before, and you believe your efforts will fail. You feel a profound sense of hopelessness, which is extremely sad. I appreciate that you're letting us look at your experience truthfully, which helps us to help you. Would you agree that this hopelessness is a potent force within you?

Ct: Yes, it is overwhelming.

Th: How about if we just make room for that fact? You believe that the future will repeat the past, and you are doomed to suffer, right?

Ct: That's true.

Use of metaphor

Th: What if this hopelessness has wrapped itself around you like a parasitic vine around an otherwise healthy tree trunk? What if the vine itself is killing the tree, sapping your energies and all possibilities for joy? What if this hopelessness is not you but a suffocating entity that has attached itself to you, believing it knows better than you? Would you be willing to consider that your certainty of failure and lack of faith in yourself dooms our attempts to succeed? How is it to hear this? How does it feel in your body to talk about this?

Ct: Strangely, seeing my hopelessness as not me gives me hope (*his voice cracks and he sheds tears*).

When this type of awareness sets in, the client's eyebrows may rise, or the eyes open wide with a startle response. People often say, "This is new!" "Why haven't I heard this before?" Carl, who was recently divorced, told me with a mix of grief and joy, having been in treatment for over a decade, "I've never had therapy like this before. It goes straight to the heart of what I've been doing to myself all my life, and it gives me hope." A visceral and life-changing perspective came into existence, allowing him to simultaneously:

- Recognize that he had built walls that were affecting our relationship. Neither of us would surmount his hopelessness unless he saw it as an illusion. He was stunned to see that he'd been pushing others away from him to keep out pain that had been too great to bear as a child. As he perceived other options, he felt empowered.

- Absorb my caring energies, fortifying his ability to face the full range of his feelings.
- Have greater faith in his ability to make new emotional and relational choices.

Therapists frequently avoid drawing attention to self-protective habits like intellectualization or detachment, fearing they will injure or offend their clients. I empathize with their hesitation as none of us wants to alienate a client. Yet, the therapist's anxiety can prevent meaningful growth. Unconsciously, we may wonder, "What feelings will swallow us up if I explore what lies beneath his words?" Our clients avoid feelings, and so do we. Therapists have told me that they have the desire and even the compulsion to change the subject when feelings rise, or they may explain the feelings away. One therapist said she'd come to me for therapy because her former therapist reinforced her intellectualization. She enjoyed their comfortable relationship, but she was avoiding rather than facing her fears of closeness.

At a major conference on countertransference, I noticed that none of the presenters mentioned anything that would trigger their countertransference in a session. Coincidentally, one of the well-known speakers had terminated therapy with a friend of mine, and he had been open enough to tell her that it was due to his countertransference. I had hoped the speakers would share some of their internal struggles and areas of avoidance to get help with my own. I empathize with the shame that makes it hard to acknowledge vulnerabilities. I was surprised to learn that I can share my fears and shortcomings with my audiences and survive.

Where to Focus First?

Let's return to Joanne, whose speech was pressured and breathless. I addressed her racing speech first, as her anxiety and compulsive talking prevented a connection between us. If she had been unable to look at me and hesitated to speak, I would focus first on shame. I wanted to draw attention to her anxiety in a way that would not feel prematurely intrusive. So, I posed questions that would invite her to discover her inner state rather than point out my observations. After Joanne interrupted me several times, we had the following exchange. Though I intended to avoid shaming, it still occurs, but hopefully to a lesser degree than without *shame sensitivity* awareness.

Th: You're talking about several important and painful things going on in your life, Joanne, and I'm so glad you're sharing them with me. I feel sadness for how overwhelming and stressful these events have been for you. I want to process and respond to all that you're feeling and experiencing. It will help me to go slowly, but I sense that something may be pressuring you to cover many things at once. Does this sound true for you too?

Ct: I'm sorry. I know I tend to talk fast. You're not the first person to tell me to slow down. *(Drawing attention to her unconscious patterns predictably arouses shame, although her temporary discomfort seems unavoidable to allow for new awareness. I offer clarification to prevent a rupture.)*

Th: I don't intend any criticism or correction, Joanne. I'm suggesting that we might offer the most help if we go slowly so we can process what you're sharing and feeling inside. There's nothing "wrong" with going fast, but we may miss something important. Does this make sense for you? How do you see it?

Ct: It's true. If I just talk, I won't get much. (*She appears to skip past this valuable realization, but there are signs it's had an effect.*) But I want you to know a few things that are going on right now.

Her words convey urgency, and I wanted to show her that she impacted me, unlike others in her life. We're negotiating between her desire to share more stories and my desire to attend to her unconscious anxiety and shame. I take her cues, validating her, and wait for opportunities to go deeper when the timing feels right.

Th: Of course! I want to hear all that is significant to you and believe that if we pursue our work, we will find the time to attend to what matters the most for you to get relief. Why don't you tell me what you want me to know now, and then let's look for a focus together?

Ct: *(She describes feeling overwhelmed by a series of family and professional events. After she became aware of her racing thoughts, her speech became less pressured.)*

Th: I'm touched by your sharing so openly with me. I can imagine myself feeling scared and overwhelmed too (*normalizing her feelings*). You've endured a lot of trauma, and I feel sad for what you've gone through. I notice that your speech has slowed down also, so I'm more able to stay with you, and you may be more comfortable too (*reinforcing her new awareness*). Since there's a world of wisdom in your body, would it be ok with you for us to see how you feel in your body as you open yourself to me in this vulnerable and courageous way?

Ct: I feel some tingling in my chest, kind of fluttering in my heart. (Her cooperative response tells us the collaborative approach is working.)

Th: I'm so glad you told me. It seems like you may have a little shortness of breath, too, would you say?

Ct: Yeah. I'm just seeing that.

Th: That's wonderful you can observe so well. Your body is giving us such vital signals, and would you agree that your thoughts sometime override distress in your body? (*She nods in agreement.*) It doesn't seem fair to you for your bodily sensations and feelings to be left unattended, would you agree?

I wait for her to consider forming an alliance with me to override her excessive verbalization and focus instead on her body-based fear, shame, and underlying feelings. My question telegraphs that there is more to her than the products of her mind. I want to transmit empathy and caring for her neglected feelings.

Ct: I've never really paid any attention to my body. I just know I want you to know my story.

Th: Yes, you want me to know what you've been through, and so do I (*validating her needs*). And I also value how you feel about what you've experienced. Very much. The sensations and feelings in your body are a gateway to the fullness of your story. They can allow both of us to connect in a way that would not be possible with words alone. This can be true for other relationships too. But I wouldn't want to proceed in this way without your agreement. How does an approach that gives attention to your body and feelings resonate for you?

Ct: Yes, I agree it could be helpful, although it scares me. (*Her rise in anxiety tells us we're entering fertile new territory.*)

Th: I can empathize with your fear, as this path would be very new for you I appreciate your telling me about your anxiety. I also wonder if you might feel shame, since trying something unfamiliar is awkward and intimidating.

I wanted my words to convey a tone of deep compassion for her lack of safety in our relationship. Joanne cried in response, and we felt the beginnings of a bond forming between us, an opening to something sweet and heartfelt.

Ct: Yes, I think that's right. I want to live differently. I don't want to feel alone, and I'll have to face my fears with you.

I mirrored Joanne's sadness for her terrible sense of aloneness and the price of her coping strategies. I believe she glimpsed the possibility of a closeness she had never known, and I sensed that my caring touched her. Her will to take emotional risks in her therapy came online.

As I mentioned, the Healing Triad came into focus during this exchange. She became AWARE of the way her compulsive speech prevented a healing relationship from forming between us. She began to absorb my COMPASSION for her suffering due to neglected anxiety and shame, rooted in past relationship traumas. She tapped into her WILL for us to connect. I recommend holding these three change elements in consciousness as we encounter treatment obstacles.

The Healing Triad helps frozen fragments of the self-start to thaw. Imagine prisoners leaving their jail cells, having been incarcerated for the crime of self-expression. The therapist and client listen for the first time to voices silenced since childhood. One of my favorite metaphors for SAGSS is the parasitic vine that sucks the life force of an otherwise healthy tree trunk, a symbol of the functional self at its core. Humiliations and deprivations cause a person to believe that their emotions and desires are wrong or selfish and will result in being stranded without human sustenance. Toxic "vines," the SAGSS, wrap their tentacles around the self, tightening a noose around its expressive, creative, and unique parts. The healthy tree trunk underneath the engulfing vines becomes hard to recognize. I hope to introduce my clients to the core parts of themselves, rich with emotion and power.

Shame Sensitivity When Shedding Light on SAGSS

Drawing attention to SAGSS (toxic shame, anxiety, guilt, and self-protective strategies) calls for attuned *shame sensitivity* to reduce the perception of criticism and increase receptivity. With practice, the therapist will find greater ease doing work with defensive processes. When a client begins to shut us out, attack or overwhelm us, we can bring compassionate awareness to these forms of self-protection and explore a more functional alternative. When the client projects that we are disapproving and rejecting, we can suggest that the client consider that we are safer and more accepting than perceived, and perhaps the client's judgments create the greatest threat! It becomes vital that we accept the client's choices about how much to explore and to risk.

You Messages

Shame sensitive interactions fortify selfhood and shaming responses weaken it. Consider the therapist's choice of words. "You" messages can be shame-inducing, yet are exceedingly common in psychotherapy when dealing with defenses. "You have changed the subject" or "You are detaching." Naturally, we will use the pronoun "you" sometimes. But when we say the client did something, we imply the client acted with conscious awareness or did something wrong. Yet, we are typically referring to unconscious processes. Who is it who detaches or diversifies? Who is it who is compliant or defiant? Another option: "Would you agree that something pulled you away from this important topic you were exploring, outside of your awareness?" Here we suggest that the client has been at the mercy of unconscious forces and conflicts. Our choice of words as we frame a comment or question, and our tone of voice, can determine whether our point will land or invite more resistance.

Building Selfhood

When we draw conclusions about the client rather than encourage self-discovery, we can unintentionally position ourselves as the superior expert, missing opportunities to strengthen selfhood. Sometimes the therapist's need for a particular outcome may create an insistence that our client uncovers or sees something. Preoccupied with our desire, we might not leave room for the client's desires. For example, we may repeatedly ask the same question, conveying we will make no room for the client to take a different direction. Clients have told me, "You've asked that question several times," or "You're repeating yourself," or "I feel like you expect an answer, and I don't know how to give it to you." An example:

Ct: You've asked me that identical question several times.

Th: Tell me about your experience.

Ct: It feels robotic. It sounds like a technique, to be honest. It doesn't feel like you're talking to me like an individual.

Th: Wow! I hadn't looked at it that way, but I can see how that would be the case. I appreciate your feedback, and to be honest, this way of questioning you doesn't feel natural to me. I value you as a unique person, and I'm sorry for giving a different impression. Could we start over?

Ct: I'd like that.

Th: Truthfully, I'm searching for ways to encourage you to connect to your feelings, as I think that's what you want and what will help you. If that's correct, do you see ways for us to open some doors together? I'd also like to hear how this exchange has been for you?

Multiple factors activate shame in therapy. When we don't try to mitigate shame, we reenact trauma. We can access feelings through a variety of routes, but I recommend the most collaborative one.

Seek Permission to Address SAGSS

To avoid shaming, we can refrain from making observations about the operation of SAGSS without explicit permission. A therapist may ask, "Do you notice you are short of breath?" or ask about the frequency of bowel movements, without ever being given explicit consent to this type of intimacy. While such inquiries contribute to healing in the right context, they can also feel invasive when the client has not granted permission to work in a particular way. Many people feel significant shame about bodily reactions that they cannot control. A person may feel mortified to disclose sudden stomach spasms or a racing heart. While these conversations provide vital information, let's be sure the client consents to them. We might ask:

> *"I've found it to be beneficial to give attention to what's happening in your body as we work. I know this is very new to most people and very personal, and I'm wondering how you would feel about this?"*

I had a conversation with some grandparents who were very disturbed that their adult son and his wife allowed their young kids to destroy others' property. The parents instantly silenced the grandparents' attempts to express their feelings. I asked if they had considered asking permission to share a few things that they thought could benefit their grandchildren, and they seemed surprised and appreciative of this idea. This same concept applies to the therapeutic relationship, though permission seeking will not achieve its desired result if it is perfunctory. Just as therapists must sometimes take "No" for an answer, the grandparents may have to live with disappointing decisions made by their son and daughter-in-law. Or, their adult children might collaborate. It's worth a discussion.

Creating Safety Requires Attunement

The willingness to observe internal processes requires safety, which we create through attuned responses to emerging phenomena. For instance, Margo opened her first session by telling me about her severe self-doubt and loathing and her desire to "see results quickly." She didn't want to repeat a drawn-out process that didn't change anything, like her prior therapy. She had concerns that she occasionally used substances as an escape mechanism. She had bouts of anxiety, fatigue, and regrets for outbursts with her boyfriend. The following describes a conflict with a female friend:

Ct: I'd taken some drugs with a group of friends. They assured me it was a safe dose. I was sitting next to a friend's husband, Bruce. I started to trip out and was having this really wild fantasy, and my mind pretty much left the room. When I came back to reality, my arm had fallen on Bruce's penis. I was horrified and quickly removed it. I stopped taking drugs altogether after that happened. I'd been given a bad batch and would not have taken something that strong. I figured my friend would understand, given the state we were both in, but she was furious and told a bunch of people about it. I couldn't believe it! (*Her voice rose, and I could feel the explosiveness inside her. Her friend was misattuned, a common theme with her mother.*) Anyway, I really don't want to go through this again.

Th: Tell me what you mean by "this?" (*I was just about to ask her about her feelings toward this friend, but her last statement made me question if I had permission to explore her feelings.*)

Ct: The incident is over. I need to move on (*she said sharply*). I've talked about my past in another therapy, and it did little. There's no point now.

I was glad I'd asked her that last question. Her shoulders and abdomen caved. She went from intensely animated to flat in a split second. Although she'd told me one of her purposes for therapy was to "recognize her emotions better," she became defiant.

Th: I hear you. You don't want to revisit a painful experience when you see nothing to gain. I certainly don't want to go anywhere you don't want to go. (*As I assured her that I would not push her, her face softened.*)

Resistance arises in a flash, and we can easily overlook it. Although she wanted to recognize her emotions better, she didn't want to explore painful feelings either. Creating this space for her to grapple with her conflict created safety and led to her next response.

Ct: I think I'm, uh, afraid. I did something this morning that scared me. (*She avoided my eyes.*)

Th: I'm glad you told me, and I can see it's hard to do. Take your time. (*She found it hard to focus, and we worked on regulating her shame and anxiety with compassionate awareness and tracking her bodily sensations.*)

Ct: I couldn't find something in my garage, and I hurled some objects against the wall. It just exploded out of me. I'm afraid of losing control of my feelings.

Th: Yes, I can see why you'd be alarmed. Has anything like that happened before? (*She said, "No."*) What do you fear you could do? What would it look like?

Ct: I just remember how my mom could go crazy, hurling her medications all over the bedroom, overturning furniture. She acted like I didn't exist. She could just do anything she felt like. And I was a little kid. (*Sadness welled up in me.*)

Th: How horrendous for you! What a shocking and terrifying experience. No wonder you see no point in making room for your feelings. Your world could collapse if you did. You'd do anything to shut down her volcanic eruptions.

Ct: I'm terrified of becoming her.

Th: That's such an important realization! I believe we could take a path that would protect you from losing control. We could stay aware of what's going on in your body. You've learned to trap your feelings inside because you don't trust them, and you've been alone with them. I think your fear spikes right before your discharge, like throwing things at the wall. We could practice regulating your anxiety so you could feel safer to recognize your feelings, which you said you wanted from our work together.

Ct: That strikes me as worthwhile, different. I'm always racing. I know I have to stop running.

Margo had never tried this specific type of shared internal focusing before. I could see my comment engendered hope as her spine straightened. She saw the possibility that both of us could bear her feelings. Although Margo had emphatically stated that she wanted "fast results," I needed to tell her the reality:

Th: Margo, you said earlier that you wanted to see results quickly, and I share your desire for fast relief. However, if we don't take the time to give attention to your fears of your feelings, we could recreate the conditions that could cause you to lose control.

Ct: I know that's right. I'm always racing and very impatient, but I'm aware I can't rush this. (*She sighed deeply and expressed relief from tension.*)

By clarifying Margo's ambivalence about facing her feelings, we discovered why she shut down and resisted therapy. Our alliance became more sturdy as she felt she'd been seen. Although she wanted to "move on," she was in the grip of her past. Becoming aware of her shame and fear of losing control was pivotal to any forward movement.

To recap the process:

1 I was about to ask Margo about her feelings toward her unforgiving friend and accuser.
2 She made a vague statement about not wanting to "do this again."
3 I did not understand the meaning of "this" and inquired about it.
4 Margo clarified that she didn't want to go further into her feelings.
5 I honored her choice.
6 She felt safer with me when I accepted her wishes.
7 She revealed her terror of losing control like her mother, and she expressed shame that she might be like her mother.
8 We reduced her shame and anxiety and established a more realistic alliance. We could not rush her therapy, as we needed to attend first to the trauma-related barriers to her feelings.

The Healing Triad—Part II

The Therapeutic Transfer of Compassion for Self

As I looked into Margo's eyes and saw her vulnerability, a state that she rarely showed, I wanted her to know that I felt pain that she had been subjected to her mother's explosive and menacing outbursts. I expressed sadness that her feelings of anger, a vital part of her, had become foreign and frightening. She met the softness in my eyes with a look that held both appreciation and suspicion. A tender feeling arose within me again, wanting to reach through her guardedness. Since her mother routinely dismissed and terrorized her, she naturally felt unsafe about drawing closer to me. If her mother showed so little interest in knowing her, why would I be any different? So she dismissed me, which seemed the safest thing to do. She smiled as she returned to the subject of her friend, but as she talked about her, her voice became sharp and staccato, and her fiery rage startled me.

Th: Did you feel that rise in emotion right then? Did you notice how your voice rose suddenly, and your tone sounded sarcastic?

Ct: I hadn't noticed. But if I reflect, I can see the anger.

This breakthrough of awareness of anger would not have occurred if my comment hadn't been immediate. Her feelings would have been repressed quickly.

Th: We see if we take our time, you can identify your anger, which will prevent you from losing control of it.

Ct: You know, my friend (*her accuser*) had a lot of trauma herself. (*Showing compassion for her friend and less splitting. She also moved away from her anger and shifted to a story about her friend's rape.*)

Th: You have compassion for your friend. You are also angry at her for judging you harshly and damaging your reputation. Your anger was strong a moment ago. Where did it go? I believe you repress anger immediately, keeping it out of awareness. Your anger then has a life of its own and lashes out in ways that damage. It needs to be recognized. I'm feeling allied with your anger because it's been thrown away. Your mother could rage uncontrollably, but you were not allowed to experience your anger at all. Do you want to make a place for it?

Ct: How do you mean?

Th: Perhaps I could demonstrate by entering the role of your anger. Would you be willing to respond to me as the voice of your anger? Would this be ok for you?

Ct: Yes.

Taking the role of anger and making it a feeling worthy of compassion

Th: (*In the voice of her anger*) I was here a minute ago. You have a habit of getting rid of me instantly.

Ct: You're right. I see no use for you. You've only been destructive in my life.

Th: I was given a bad rap. You're right that I feel impulses to destroy, but that doesn't mean that I will destroy in reality. I've been living inside you for years, and I've rarely lost control. There's a difference between a feeling and an action. Your mother acted out her rage and terrified you, but I'm not her. I have other ways to express myself.

Ct: Like what?

Th: I'm just an energy that wants to move through your body. I just want you to notice what I feel like in your body without restraint.

> Do you think I'm an accident of nature? Why should I be banished from existence? I'm here for a purpose. When you're hurt, my angry impulses want to protect you, but I will not act out like your mother. I have other options if you will allow me to come into awareness. You will feel more whole. But if you turn away from me, you abandon a vital part of yourself. Would you be willing to treat me as a friend and ally and show interest in me instead?

Since Margo had many successes in her life, she had minimized the cost of repressing and judging her feelings. But when I tuned into the constant tautness in Margo's muscles, her distrusting look, and her readiness to find fault and pull away at any moment, we could both sense the toll on her body and spirit. She was unable to feel secure in any of her relationships.

From "Change Partners" by Stephen Stills (1971):
Please then remember
And don't get too close to one special one
He will take your defenses and run
So we change partners
Time to change partners
You must change partners
Again

Unnecessary losses that multiply over the years, involving friendships, spouses, careers, and families, create a wasteland! The original traumas inflicted on a child spawn subsequent losses, evoking great tenderness in me. This compassionate feeling may slip imperceptibly from my body into my client's. Many therapists know this experience, though they may not name it. I call this phenomenon the TTCS, the Therapeutic Transfer of Compassion for Self. I am moved when I witness this transfer, even though it may be fleeting and will need to be reactivated many times in the course of treatment.

Resistance to the Transference of Compassion

Rene had a flourishing career and was now in her mid-sixties. She'd broken up with Andy, a man she'd dated for a couple of years. He adored her, but she recoiled from his readiness to please her. She saw his compliant habits as a deal-breaker.

Ct: All the men I've fallen in love with betrayed or abandoned me. With Andy, I'm afraid I might be passing on the best relationship opportunity I may ever have. Andy drove me here, and he's in the waiting room. He'd do anything for me. That's what bothers me about him. He's too accommodating. My friends and former therapist want me to be with him. You probably feel the same way.

Th: Tell me how you hope I can help you? (*I hope to bring her desires to consciousness and step outside her projection of will that it is me who wants something.*)

Ct: I'm terrified I will spend my life alone. I'm not getting younger. This problem remains after years of therapy.

Th: So you're afraid you could be making the wrong decision if you leave Andy? And you won't have such a good opportunity again? Are you saying you want me to help you to make a sound decision?

Ct: I think that's right. I can't trust myself.

Th: It's a shame that you don't trust your perceptions or your feelings, which may have been brushed aside over the years. You manage so many areas of your life with great competence, but helplessness sets in when it comes to your personal needs. After all these years of serial relationships, many of them heartbreaking, we might wonder if something operates inside you that keeps a healthy relationship perpetually out of reach? Consciously you want closeness, but unconsciously some force keeps you confused and disconnected from what you feel and desire. If you want, we could work together to strengthen these internal signals.

Ct: You'd think I would have achieved that by now. But in the meantime, I'm afraid I'm making a big mistake by pushing Andy away. (*She wants me to guide her decision with Andy rather than grapple with an internal conflict.*)

Th: I understand your concern. You don't know if you're listening to the healthiest part of you. I don't know either. It would seem risky to make decisions before you clarify the feelings within yourself.

Ct: See, you are telling me to stay with him. You're just like everyone else. (*She projected her will that I want her to stay with Andy.*)

Th: You've sought therapy with me to get a sense of direction. You're raising some excellent questions. Who is it that makes your relationship decisions? So far, you say it hasn't been working out. Until your feelings get clarified, your relationship decisions will be on shaky ground. You are capable of good decisions, and it won't help you for me to direct you.

Ct: You're right. That's true.

Th: I empathize with your suffering due to profound fears of remaining alone and never finding a good enough partner.

Ct: I'm not aware of being in pain.

Awakening compassion for the suffering caused by unconscious patterns can be challenging with clients who have long histories of self-dismissal. In a subsequent session, I addressed her habit of ignoring internal distress signals, which left her unprotected. We also discussed her intense judgments of herself and the men she dated.

Ct: I've been catching myself in the act of judging Andy and myself several times in the past week. (*I saw this as a positive sign of a therapeutic alliance, but her awareness of a problem doesn't mean she will attend to it.*)

Th: So you've been noticing and interrupting these automatic attacks on you and Andy?

Ct: Oh, I wouldn't say I'm interrupting. (*She confirms her passivity around the self-flagellating part of her. Nothing will change if this passivity remains.*) I've been conscious of them. I would say I step in and just say, "Oh, there I go again." And then I do see that, and it's tied into a suspicious thing toward Andy. Suspicious, critical. And that's the kind of consciousness I've had since I've been talking to you recently.

Awareness of a defense without the will to attend to it

We can appreciate her growing awareness of her judgmental mind. However, she does not yet have the will to treat herself differently. I must bring the absence of will to care for herself, and its consequences, to consciousness before a pattern shift can occur. Her suspiciousness arises from her fear of closeness, and alarms go off when a potential mate comes too near.

Th: That's great that you're becoming aware of this deep habit of finding fault and deficiency, which leads to suspicion and loneliness. But you don't interrupt it, as you would if you saw that your granddaughter was doing something that would hurt herself. I'm sure you would go toward her immediately and do everything you could to relieve her suffering.

Ct: Yes. I can do that with my granddaughter. I can do that with a pet. I can do that with adult friends.

Th: I have no doubt! But when it comes to you, you can be aware of an internal harming force but not intervene.

Ct: I don't think I've reached that point, Susan. I don't think I'm aware that my criticism toward myself causes me pain.

Th: Oh, that's a great observation.

Ct: It's just something I'm doing, and I'm not conscious of it hurting me. It's just who I am. And I'm always going 90 miles an hour.

Th: Rushing past your best interests. Yet, I've seen your pain firsthand.

Ct: You have?

Th: Yes. I can even sometimes feel it in my own body.

Ct: That's intense, and you know what? I believe you because I trust you.

Th: I'm glad you trust me. I want you to feel that. I sense your pain from the expression on your face when you say, "I'm a failure," I see the pain of shame on your face.

A child needs a parent to help her identify what she feels. Rene had little mirroring or caring attention as a child. She learned to disguise her needs and feelings, trying to be her father's ideal. She deflects my comments, pushing away closeness.

Ct: Yes, I think that most people that are productive would get frustrated. (*She generalizes and rationalizes the internal attacker that lives inside her.*)

Th: I'm speaking about the part that says, "I have failed. I couldn't even get a relationship right." This part puts you down mercilessly.

Ct: Ah. Yeah. I think there's a critical connection to that because that's what I do to the men in my life that I want to be close to. That's real, and they're innocent. I find myself always apologizing the next day. That's not healthy. I've been talking to a lot of different men, just figuring out who I want to go out with, and what I want to do, but also consciously watching my behavior and my words, and then my apologies, and I'm saying to myself, "This is a pattern I need to stop. I need to clarify where this is coming from and why it keeps coming like Tourette's."

Th: So, you recognize that this judging part hurts them, and you want to stop doing that. But you're not aware that it inflicts pain on you too. Your disconnection from yourself can't be ignored if anything is to change. You've learned to ignore your suffering.

Ct: No. I would love to resonate with that one. I would love to connect those dots. I think that could be very helpful. I understand intellectually what I'm doing and how it could hurt me, but I don't feel it. I don't get it. (*I feel very saddened. She can't have self-compassion if she doesn't experience the pain caused by her defensive habits. I attempt to work with her denial.*)

Th: Would you be coming to me, Rene, if you weren't suffering from intense anxiety, dread, and condemnation of yourself and others?

Ct: I'm coming because—you know, I'm coming because I keep myself at a distance, and I'm critical to men, and I'd like to be in a loving, long-term relationship. I'd like to have another 10, 15, 20 years of history with one man, and give him love and allow his love to penetrate. And I'm conflicted about why I don't understand my feelings better. I don't even know if I'm not missing this guy that I was with because I'm sick and I'm detached from my emotions and feelings. Or is he just the wrong guy? Maybe I never met the right guy. (*Externalization of the problem.*) I'm conflicted, I'm confused, and yes, there is some suffering along the way. You feel as though you should be in a straitjacket emotionally. You can't move in the right direction. You can't. And I'm results-oriented. I've got so much in my life to be grateful for. This piece is so elusive and confusing.

Th: I'm glad you recognize your internal suffering. How does it feel to see these internal forces that inflict pain on you? (Attempting to increase her awareness of suffering and help her to feel it in the body.)

Projection

Ct: And I have a strong feeling that you have 100% awareness that they cause me suffering.

Th: I only know what you tell me, Rene. You describe your distress, but you sadly don't register pain or suffering, which blocks compassion for yourself. I'm in touch with my compassion for you and desire for your happiness, but nothing will shift if you don't experience it, would you agree? (*I return the projection and highlight the reality of the consequences of her denial and rationalization.*)

Ct: Well, I'm glad that you want that for me. I really appreciate that. Ok. Alright. So, let's get into the suffering. What about this suffering that I have?

Th: You want to go through life without overwhelming fear and dread, and you want to share your life with someone you love. These longings have eluded you, and you keep the pain out of awareness.

Ct: That makes sense. I get that. Mm-hmm. Well, yes. I am a woman who would like to have a loving, connected, intimate relationship that's ongoing. I've had a struggle with that. Do I think it's tied into how I treat myself, perceive myself, and the end result causes me suffering, and hurts people around me, hurt myself by being alone? Yes. Yes. (*She is aware but detached from herself.*)

Th: Loving is kind. Loving is forgiving and compassionate.

Ct: I have those words all over my house. Yeah. That's what it is, and I can be that with friends, clients, employees, girlfriends, children, and grandchildren. I can't seem to be that way with any consistency with a personal relationship.

Th: What about the relationship with you? (*Will she show compassion for herself?*)

Ct: And that's a good question. So, why doesn't it register with me? Because I can take it. I can handle it. I'm not going to leave me. It's physically impossible. I've got too many things to do to let it register or slow me down, and too many responsibilities to too many people. I'm trying to just throw something out for why I don't connect to that. I'm sure it's real.

Th: It might be why you don't have what you want. A habit of denial doesn't allow you to see that you are suffering due to a lack of relationship to your feelings.

Ct: The only way to create a shift from this life that is causing me suffering is to have an awareness that I am suffering and to allow myself to feel that suffering?

Th: Exactly! And to care about your suffering. As I see it, that's the only way forward. (*I hope to transfer my caring energies to her.*)

Tai Chi with the Judging, Indifferent Force

I don't want to go up against the judging force, a learned, unconscious, inherently protective strategy that creates distance. Closeness equals failure and abandonment in her unconscious mind. I want to hold the judge in my arms, strange as that sounds, for it is frantic, lost, and poignantly misguided. I want to gently illuminate it, as light penetrates that which is dark and destructive.

Ct: Yes. I see I've had a pattern for years of being critical, sabotaging, pushing away, and leaving the men that are good to me. And I chased those who have been poor to me, bad to me, mean to me, not there for me. That causes me suffering.

Th: It's great you see that so clearly. So, you don't let in the good?

Ct: Right. I don't. That's why I'm still single.

Th: Wow! This comment says it all. You're talking about a long-standing, habitual pattern that pushes away potential mates by focusing on their faults. And the judging part of you shows up like an oracle that embodies the ultimate and absolute truth (*like her father*). When that whole system is operating, there's no separation between you and it. Its voice booms, "Truth is speaking! This man has flaws, and you must not tolerate flaws. Nor can you tolerate your feelings toward him. Get far away from him and your feelings as fast as you can." The oracle takes you over a cliff, where you will perpetually be alone, feel unloved, dissatisfied, and unfulfilled. Nevertheless, the oracle proclaims the absolute truth, and it's hard to see that you can't trust it to guide you properly.

Ct: I shouldn't get close because now, all of a sudden, these men have been destroyed in my view. They are not someone I should be with because they have all these flaws.

Th: Yes! That's the oracle. It gobbles up people and relationships. It gobbles you up. It can gobble me up. It can gobble up the man who is with you. And then your suffering continues, and it's done its thing. And then you'll say nothing has shifted after years of working on this problem. Well, it can't shift when you tie yourself to this oracle, this—

Ct: Force. This force. This force is so certain in its judgments. Yeah. I'm so positive.

Th: This part is absolute. And you identify with that part.

Ct: Yes. So, then I saw all of his flaws from this oracle of truth. It was so true and it was saying to me, "Now it's ok to let go of him (*her last boyfriend*) completely."

Th: Right. You've followed the oracle for a long time.

Ct: I'm sick of this oracle. I'm sick of this oracle.

Th: So, there is something in you that lives outside of the oracle, right? There is something in you that is separate from this oracle?

Ct: You're very good at keeping me on task. Yes. There is something other than just that oracle. Yes.

Metaphors often become lastingly meaningful. Their symbolism sticks in a way that ideas wouldn't otherwise. Because they are quickly understood and absorbed, metaphors do not trigger shame. Rene would reference the oracle repeatedly in future sessions. As she considers separating from the "oracle" that makes secure attachment impossible, she begins to recognize anxiety in her body. Rene discovers that she fears separating from the behavior that pleased her parents, who idealized love. She connects to the pain of seeking idealized love for the first time.

Ct: The oracle is so incredibly contradictory of everything that I want, which then continues the cycle of confusion. There's no shift from that behavior, from that oracle that has control over me, but because there's still a piece of me, I think, that believes something that was ingrained in me as a child, as a baby, that love knows, love will come when it's right, and love is all-knowing, and love conquers all. My parents idealized love. I hold onto the idea that I should remove myself from someone with flaws. That sign means that I haven't met the right person. And that keeps me on this thing. It does.

Th: Right. A hamster on a treadmill.

Ct: Yes. Yeah. And there are these patterns, and then when these men fall in love with me, bye-bye. All these flaws come up. And if the guy is really tough to get close to, wow, I'm in love. It's a sad way to live. (*If a man were to embrace her, what must be wrong with him?*)

Th: Do you feel the sadness, the pain?

Ct: The fact that this pattern has a hold on me is very painful.

Th: Tell me more how you feel this pain? Could we stay with your pain?

Ct: Andy was probably, of every man who's been with me, the most unconditionally loving, and I have more criticism of him than I've had with any man before. I feel the sadness now (*her eyes well up*).

As her denial and minimization of her suffering break down, Rene sheds tears. She recognizes the cost of her distancing behaviors and begins to feel the pain they've caused. The TTCS sprouts tender new roots.

The Healing Triad—Part III

The Will to Feel and Connect Deeply to Others

In DEFT, we hope to awaken the desire to achieve the highest quality relationships possible, involving emotional attunement to self and others and refined relationship skills. The therapist models and raises awareness of central elements in a secure attachment. When a client communicates empathy for the first time in significant relationships, we know this shift is occurring. Mobilization of the will to experience feelings and draw closer to others requires courage. The client must step outside a lifetime of conditioning onto a tight wire suspended over the unknown. Emotional truth is terrifying, especially if we're meeting it for the first time. Who will catch us if we fall and can't get up again?

Most people believe they know what they feel and don't see a need to feel more. People are typically amazed to discover otherwise. Humans can't accurately interpret emotional signals without knowing how to read their bodies. Unconscious shame, anxiety, and guilt often block the passageways to unconscious feelings. Without the will, we will not ask ourselves the vital questions: "What are my feelings right now?" "How do I feel toward you (or another specific person)?" "Do I recognize the range of my feelings, or do I reduce them to a shadow of their true dimensions?" Emotional connection to the therapist relies on these questions and their answers. The will to feel and connect shifts the therapeutic partnership into a new gear. This same occurs with ones' spouse, child, or friend. A real response replaces a programmed reaction. We feel life in place of deadness, surprise instead of predictability, revelation rather than confusion.

How do we know when the will is active? A person might say, "Let's do it!" Or "I don't want to live this way anymore. I'm willing to try something new." Will is implicit when unconscious emotional memories bubble to the surface. One woman who had been unable to remember any positive experiences with her abusive mother suddenly recalled, "I can remember my mother's voice, clear as a bell, 'Joanie, it's time to get up.' That tone in her voice was how I could feel her love." In another instance, a man's will allowed him to face that he'd gone into medicine solely because his father was a doctor and wanted him to follow in his footsteps. He'd never seen this before. He'd unconsciously left his talents and passions by the wayside to please his father. When he heard himself speak this truth, enormous pain engulfed him. Afterwards, he felt energy rise from his torso, pulling his spine upwards, as a triumphant feeling filled his body. He could declare his truth and challenge his father.

We see evidence that the will is online when the client volunteers risky and revealing information. We witness the presence of will when we hear comments such as, "I just noticed a jabbing pain in my neck," or "This reminds me of the time Dad threw a shoebox at me. I'm starting to feel heat in my chest." When an elderly gentleman who routinely avoided eye contact began to cry without covering his face, his will triumphed. These acts of will are brave and moving.

Michael was the most shame-based person I've ever treated. Extreme forms of self-hatred, self-defiling, and self-disgust overshadowed his considerable charms and artistic talents. His deceased father had been violent, beating him with belts and bats. He should have been criminally charged for his abuses. His mother ran from reality and dragged Michael thoughtlessly from state to state. His parents systematically ignored this boy's longings for stability and safety. What he wanted didn't matter, and soon he paid no attention to his desires either. He acted out the rage he couldn't own. As an adolescent, he and his closest friend beat each other for fun every day after school. It is such a great injustice when victims of abuse and neglect are retraumatized by turning rage against themselves.

Despite his detachment, social anxiety, defiance, and sarcastic teasing, Michael and I managed to enter profound emotional territory together. But, he did not extinguish his habits of hiding and dismissing himself quickly. After a period of progress, when I was feeling hopeful for him, he suddenly pulled back. He didn't feel like coming to therapy. I was shocked. This could be his last session. An equally strong voice told me, "Don't make this session about your hopes that Michael stay. He will want to continue, or he won't. Explore what's happening and respect his will!" It would have been easy to internalize Michael's sense of stagnation and hopelessness through projective identification. Or, I could try to persuade him to keep going, but Michael would have rejected any such attempts, as he was a master debater. Our exchange went like this:

Ct: I've been telling myself lately that I don't want to come here, and I'm not sure it's because I don't want to come here or because I'm starting to wonder if I'm going to or can gain much more.

His openness is a sign of our alliance. The fact that he's sharing truthfully with me is positive. But within me, there's a place that says, "I have nothing more to give him." Both of us have doubts. But it's my will to override that part of me that is resigning.

Th: I'm glad you told me, and I appreciate your openness. May I ask, is there anything you are hoping for at this point in your therapy? You said you wondered if you could gain more? Is there more you want to gain? (*Reinforcing the significance of Michael's desires and agency.*)

Ct: I don't know. Lately, I have limited, miniature purposes, projects, aspirations, but any one of them could dissipate, and it just wouldn't make much difference. I feel kind of lost.

Th: So you don't feel connected to any desires for yourself?

Ct: No. Well, I mean, I am, but I don't feel passionate or strongly, really, about any of it. I mean, I don't know. I mean, I like the comfortable part where I don't have to risk intimate relationships at this time.

Attachment deprivation drives his recurrent depression. However, he would crush any argument that relationships have value. He's tried to escape intimacy through addictions, and he believes his ego-syntonic, distancing mechanisms serve him.

Ct: And, I don't know, it just feels like I'm keeping time. Going nowhere, just going through the motions. Daily basis. And nothing much has much meaning. And I know that's a very depressing approach. (*I hear an opening. A part of him is protesting his depression, and I encourage that voice.*)

Th: Why do you say your approach is depressing, Michael?

Ct: Well, that's a big question. It might be tough to put my finger on that (*hiding his suffering with vagueness*).

His father's beatings and his mother's passivity stunted his yearnings. Our best shot is to raise awareness of his passivity and vagueness with tenderness and shame sensitivity.

Th: I see how hard it is, Michael, to bring into focus anything you want for yourself. Your desires disappear into a cloud of fuzziness, which I imagine is about sustaining that safe place you described, saying you liked not having to risk intimate relationships. I also hear that you think your approach is depressing, and I sense disappointment about your therapy as though you hoped for something more?

Ct: (*He pushes back.*) I don't think I'm going to achieve a goal, and I don't want to achieve a goal. I don't want a goal. I don't want any goals. I mean, I have these projects that I hope I'll benefit from later on, but as far as a goal, I don't have a goal.

Th: I completely accept this, Michael. You surely don't need to have any goals to please me. I'm here to serve you and not the other way around. It's not surprising that you would feel that you're not getting anywhere in your therapy since you have nowhere you want to get.

I pass the baton to Michael. If he seeks nothing, he will get nothing. I try to dispel magical thinking about my powers or intentions to make decisions for him, as his parents did.

Ct: No. There is nowhere to "get." (*He smiles with faint recognition that he holds the reins of his treatment.*)

Th: Yeah. Because if we don't have our eye on someplace you want to go, we're not going to go anywhere. Make sense?

Ct: Yeah. I don't have my eye on someplace I want to go. In a specific sense, anyway. I mean, I know when I come here, I'm supposed to have a goal. A goal of therapy. Well, I don't have a goal. I don't want a goal.

This exchange illustrates the defense of the "projection of will." Michael projects that I am pushing him toward a direction he doesn't want. I must not fall into this role. He believes I want him to have a goal, but he remains unaware of what he wants. I need to hold this tragedy in my consciousness, or I could give up with him. It would be easy to feel discounted and discouraged. Instead, I am committed to assist his self-exploration.

Th: How do you feel about the fact that you don't have a goal?

Ct: Well, life makes more sense when you have a goal. You know? Life is—it fills a sense of purpose. It's a better feeling than not—than to be— (*We hear his dissatisfaction with the absence of desires.*)

Th: So, it's an unpleasant feeling when you have nothing you're striving to achieve?

Ct: Yeah, it's unpleasant. It lacks pleasantness. It's not painful in itself, but it's just that there's a lack—kind of an empty, lack of pleasantness. Pleasantness missing. I'm not—and I'm not on the fence about whether I want a long-term relationship or not. I guess I've just decided that I don't want a long-term relationship or intimate relationship, and I don't care.

Th: You speak of emptiness, and there's a sense of resignation. And you find yourself in harm's way (*Michael had told me that his girlfriend's husband could potentially kill him*), and yet you don't seem moved by your suffering. (*He pauses for an extended period.*)

Ct: I'm a failure as a father, making it impossible for me to have any happiness. My daughter is an addict. My son is struggling. If they go down, I go down.

Facing his guilt for having left his children at a young age is unbearable. Instead of facing the pain of his guilt, making reparations and meaning of his life, self-punishment paralyzes him. His guilt needs to be faced, tolerated, and transcended if he can become an emotionally available father and positive role model for his grown children. At this moment, my intuition guides me to work on his shattered sense of self and intrinsic unworthiness before tackling his unprocessed guilt. I wish to raise awareness of his crippling rationale for resignation.

Th: Seems to me that there's always a reason why you can't be happy. I admit you've got a couple of good reasons, but even when your kids show signs of improvement, your investment in yourself is meager. Out of your guilt, you put yourself in harm's way and abandon yourself. Your unconscious mind uses your past failures as a club, and probably doesn't want you to keep benefiting from therapy. How can we create anything good for you when you believe you're worthless and must be denied happiness?

Ct: Yeah.

Th: Something ties you to this state of deprivation, not allowing you to dream about what you want in life. (*He pauses a long time to reflect. However, his self-sabotaging habits fight back.*)

Ct: I don't believe in happiness (*said with disdain and cynicism*). I don't believe in metamorphosis.

An internal battle ensues, and immediately after his comment, his anxiety rises. He sighs deeply and rubs his neck. His healthy part slips in, and he describes the metamorphosis he has already experienced in therapy.

Ct: I don't believe some metamorphosis is going to happen. I mean, being comfortable around people has been a major goal for my whole life. And, since I've been coming here, I'm much more comfortable and confident around people than I was. And I guess I didn't look any further than that. I didn't look beyond that because that's what I wanted. That's what plagued me. That's the biggest success I've had here.

Th: That's something you wanted and achieved. A big accomplishment! You've been on a plateau, since you don't want anything for yourself right now. When you allow yourself to have desires, they become possible. When you shut down your desires, everything stagnates.

As we go forward, we'll see the three forces of the Healing Triad merge (Awareness of SAGSS, Compassion for Self and Will) and create a radical internal shift:

Ct: Yeah. I was just singing that song today. "Is that all there is?" (*He implies he wants more for himself, but he slumps and detaches. I decide to risk sharing what is going on inside me, as I sense the abyss beckoning to both of us.*)

Th: Michael, I feel lost in a fog of vagueness, confusion, and a smokescreen. I think something in you distances automatically from closeness as a survival mechanism. Trauma caused you to fear the feelings that relationships arouse. I don't think you do any of this purposefully. I've no doubt something is trying to protect you, but I also flounder, wondering how to be useful to you when you seem far away. This realization deeply saddens me.

Here I express compassion for the enormous cost of his distancing mechanisms, which prevents me from helping him. Michael's self-reflective capacity engages. He becomes silent and deeply thoughtful during a long pause. Sadness shows on his face. A sigh and deep respiration signal a rise of anxiety, a promising sign his detachment is dissipating as feelings become activated. Soon after, he recalls significant childhood memories, an indicator his will to reveal and connect are awakening.

Ct: Distancing from closeness. That's my M.O. (modus operandi).

Th: Yeah. You said earlier, "We're never going to figure me out," as though you don't want to be known. (*A state shift occurs as an unconscious memory floats to the surface. His desperate attempts to distance from the pain of relationships started very early.*)

Ct: My eighth-grade teacher told me that. He couldn't figure me out, and he didn't think that I could be figured out, something like that.

Th: This has been going on for a long time.

Ct: Yeah. I remember in fourth or—it was sixth grade. There was this guy—ugly guy. What an ugly guy! Very muscular. He worked out a lot. We would periodically beat each other to a pulp. Not in the face, but just start throwing punches at each other as hard as we could to see how much we could take. We weren't mad at each other. It was a game.

Th: And what made you think of that?

Ct: Well, you said I must be trying to see how much I can take, punching I can take, or something like that. The picture flashed in my head. (*I remember speaking about putting himself in harm's way.*)

Th: Yeah. You have a tragic tolerance for suffering.

Ct: Tolerance for suffering. That's my survival mechanism, to build up a great tolerance for suffering because I can't change. I never affected any change. I had no power to go on the offense with my father, or no ability to convince my mother, and—

Th: Convince her of?

Ct: I don't know. Convince her that something was wrong, and I needed to—that something was wrong.

Th: That you needed help. (*Acknowledging his healthy dependency longings.*)

Ct: Yeah. So, the only strength I had was how much pain I could absorb.

Th: Well, I think you took all that rage that you never could process with your parents and took it out on this kid and yourself.

Ct: Yeah.

Th: Rage consumed you.

Ct: Yeah.

Th: Because you felt powerless. But that was then, Michael. Why would the same apply today?

Ct: Because that's the program, that's the plan.

Th: Well, that's the program that you relied upon.

Ct: That's the survival plan.

Th: Yeah. It was necessary for your survival then to find an outlet for your rage with this other kid, to conceal your feelings, and to hurt yourself. I agree that was a survival plan that was resourceful at that time. But it's heartbreaking to me, thinking of you relying on a plan that a child devised, a strategy that leaves you feeling empty. A plan that leaves you feeling lost. (*I'm cautious not to mention his lost relationships, which could trigger argumentativeness. I want to stay close to his immediate experience.*)

Ct: Every time I let down my guard, I get hurt.

Th: Could we also say that you can't make sound judgments when your feelings do not inform you? Could we say that these walls keep you disconnected from your feelings and other people? Including me?

This last statement has a profound impact, pointing to the reality that our relationship paid a price when there was distance between us. Vagueness and detachment sabotage emotional closeness. Will Michael care enough about our relationship and himself to find the will to move past his protective strategies? He has denied his need for a relationship. Will Michael let himself need one with me? He suddenly moved out of his slumped position and sat forward. He tried to deny the fact that his defenses have consequences to our relationship.

Ct: I'm trying to think. Who am I disconnected from that I should be more connected to?

Th: Well, Michael, I'm looking at the way that you disconnect from us with vagueness and indifference toward yourself, and therefore your therapy stalls. I genuinely accept your choices here, even though I feel sad about them.

Ct: I'm not hiding any feelings. I'm not—I don't think I deny any feeling. I may be reluctant to get your point.

Th: Perhaps I missed something, but I'm not aware you've expressed any feelings or desires, Michael. When I hear that you feel empty and your life is flat, but you're "fine," I feel confused. I hear that you're suffering but have no choice but to suffer because your kid is suffering—and your kid has always been suffering—so that means you have no choice but to be suffering. But you say you're fine. You say you don't want anything for yourself that you're not getting anything from therapy, and there's a sense of disappointment in that. And yet, you don't want anything. You smile now. Do you have some feelings?

Ct: It reminds me of a scene in a movie I saw with a psychiatrist.

Th: What are you feeling?

Ct: I imagined how frustrating it must be for you for me to put out a lot of confusion and smokescreens.

Th: Perhaps I feel frustrated when I can't help you, but mostly, I feel sad. It's sad to me that you accept so little for yourself.

Ct: I settled. I've always seen happiness as me being able to be comfortable around people, and I'm a lot more comfortable around people since I've been in therapy.

Th: Yes! And that was a goal you set for yourself and achieved. I congratulate you. But then, when you said you haven't been getting anywhere here for a while, I asked, "Well, what is your goal? "You answered, "I don't have a goal. I don't want a goal. But not having a goal isn't a pleasant feeling, but I don't want one." So, I guess you let yourself achieve so much, and then that's it.

Ct: I never thought past that. That's all I ever wanted. But life goes on.

Th: Is that all you want now? (*Big question. This is where the rubber meets the road. Will he declare a desire or settle as he has all his life?*)

Ct: You seem to think that there's this intimate emotional connection that I could have with my kids or people that I love if I was willing to work for that. (*His comment fascinates me. I never said any of this! Again he projected his desires onto me, and he cannot hear his own voice.*)

Th: I don't think I said that, Michael. I did say that I think you fear the feelings that come up in relationships.

Ct: Well, that's how I'm interpreting it. You seem to think there's a more intimate way of life. (*Again, he projects onto me his longing for intimacy rather than own the longing inside himself.*)

Th: You know, your mind keeps wanting to put this back on me about what I think.

Ct: It is what you think.

Th: Seems to me that what matters is what you want in therapy, what you want in your life. Because so long as you don't want for yourself, you won't have for yourself. You know? There's no way I can help you. (*Here, I raise his awareness of the terrible cost of projecting his desires onto me and disowning them within himself. He sentences himself to an empty life. He makes a significant shift as he faces reality.*)

Ct: I think I'm so wrapped up in everyday life that I don't even look at what I want out of relationships, what could be a better relationship, a more satisfying connection with someone.

Th: Or a better existence.

Ct: A better existence. Suffering is normal.

Michael had never allowed himself to acknowledge his longings for intimacy and attachment, having suffered unbearably in two failed marriages and a lifetime of emotional isolation from his family. As he notices his indifference toward his desires, he sits forward and is more self-reflective and engaged. Hope and will become revived, and he realizes he can potentially separate from the self-punishing force. I feel moved.

Th: So, you said you got some guy to beat you up as a kid and put yourself in a position with this woman where her husband could kill you. Is that another way you could unconsciously engineer getting beaten up again? And if there isn't somebody out there to beat you up, you have an internal abuser who can do it for you. I don't know if I need to recount all the ways.

Ct: No. You don't need to (*he says softly, with a wry sadness*).

Th: But there are a lot of them, would you agree?

Ct: Yes, I would agree.

Th: This makes me feel so sad. You haven't deserved this much suffering. At the same time, you've had many successes in treatment—conquering your social avoidance, working through your grief over losing your wife and no longer being disabled by depression. And there's also the monumental accomplishment of staying sober for the past 15 years! These were all goals that you set for yourself. You've demonstrated that when you want something for yourself and work to achieve it, things get better for you (*emphasizing the power of his desire*). Today your needs can have an impact! But, when you give up on yourself, then nothing improves.

Ct: Well, I don't know if there is a butterfly, but I could take your word and put my faith in you. (*He proposes to take my word rather than own his accomplishments and ability to progress. Does he dare to hope? I highlight the objective reality.*)

Th: How about if we look at objective reality together? Is it not a butterfly if you say you've had terrible social anxiety, and now you are comfortable around people—is that not a butterfly?

Ct: That's a butterfly.

Th: Inside of you?

Ct: Yeah.

Th: Ok. So, are you saying that there can't be other butterflies? You've demonstrated that you can grow, and you can find new ways of being that break the "program" given to you as a child.

Ct: (*Michael suddenly detaches again, slumping and deflated, and mounts line after line of resistance.*)

Th: Do you notice the shift from hopefulness to hopelessness? Is this what you want?

Ct: Is there any other way to be? (*He then rationalizes that genetic factors and being a man prohibit him from connecting with his feelings. He becomes argumentative.*)

Th: You've successfully connected with your feelings in treatment before.

Ct: That's true and it was always a struggle. But it relieved my tension afterwards, and I felt relaxed and good. I haven't experienced this relief today. Maybe I am afraid of my emotions. I guess I depended on this Plan B program for so long, this survival program, that I never learned Plan A. I never learned to have a feeling, and if it was uncomfortable to stay with it and ride it out and deal with it and process it and be done with it. I never learned that (*from either parent*). I've done that here. You know? It's like pulling teeth to get me to do it, and I have had an enormous reluctance to do it. And that muscle's really weak. Atrophied.

Th: How do you feel about that atrophied muscle?

Ct: Well, it's part of the hand that I'm dealt. (*Michael again takes the passive, defeated position to avoid his fears of feeling.*)

Th: It seems to me, Michael, that your feelings unconsciously shut down to survive, and I deeply empathize with your attachment to these protective mechanisms. Most unfortunately, a wall arises around you that imprisons you. And, of course, it feels empty to live inside those walls. So, life is going to feel flat. You know? It's an absence of feeling. Empty.

Ct: My macho exterior can't be looking silly. (*Michael reveals that he feels shame, embarrassment and vulnerability when he exposes feelings.*)

Th: How sad that a force attacks and shames you when you take a step toward freedom. You've learned to link pleasure to pain.

Michael becomes reflective for an extended time and surprises me with the emergence of a renewed therapeutic alliance. His will comes online, and he expresses a new engagement in therapy.

Ct: What exercise, when I leave here, could I do until I come back next time? I mean, I don't want to live afraid of my feelings. I don't want to have a part of me that I live with that makes me scared. Next time, I will come to exercise!

Th: Well, it sounds like you found a goal, huh?

The future of Michael's treatment stood in the balance during this session. The outcome could have gone either way. True to his word, Michael returned the next week, and for many months after that, and exercise, he did! Following a period of profound work that included processing his rage toward his mother, Michael decided to drive a long distance to visit his mother over the holidays. He habitually stayed away from her, but he'd turned a corner in therapy and began to feel generous toward her. He painted her entire apartment! During this visit, he had a remarkable encounter with his brother too. His brother used to beat him violently as a child, following in his father's footsteps, and Michael avoided him for many years. He was amazed that he could relax on the sofa with his brother, and his brother laid his head on his lap! Michael initiated a conversation about their childhood memories. Together they attempted to make sense of their shared nightmares.

At moments like this, I feel intensely grateful for the privilege of being a therapist. When we witness a birth, or more accurately a rebirth, of parts of the self that have been long dead, we rejoice. A thief had robbed Michael of his life force, and I cheered as he reclaimed the treasure that belonged to him. The Healing Triad allowed him to see the following with new eyes:

Awareness:

1 He had learned to bully his feelings out of existence.
2 His feelings rightfully belonged to him.
3 He was dying on the vine without the life-giving nutrients of his emotions, essential to human connection.

Compassion for Self:

4 He recognized the tragic losses resulting from self-harming behaviors and emotional deprivation.
5 He experienced that I cared deeply about his suffering, and then he cared.

Will:

6 As he began to care about himself, the will to give attention to his desires and needs rose up within him. He would no longer settle for settling.

The will is the determination to feel our feelings and surmount any obstacle that blocks them. Will is an unstoppable force that allows us to express ourselves and to connect authentically to others. Will relies on courage and love. Will shows up when oppressed parts of the self suddenly declare, "I exist. I have rights. No one will silence my voice again!" When the will to make space for the buried parts of the self appears, I want to jump for joy!

References

Alpert M.C. (1992). Accelerated empathic therapy: A new short-term dynamic psychotherapy. *International Journal of Short-Term Psychotherapy*, 7 (3), 133-156.

Couglin Della Selva, P. (2001). *Intensive short-term dynamic psychotherapy: Theory and technique*. Wiley.

Davanloo, H. (2000). *Intensive short-term dynamic psychotherapy*. Wiley.

Ecker, B., Ticic, B., and Hulley. (2012). *Unlocking the emotional brain*. Routledge.

Fosha, D. (2000). *The transforming power of affect*. Basic Books.

Frederickson, Jon. (2013). *Co-creating change*. Seven Leaves Press.

Frederickson, Jon. (2021). *Co-creating safety*. Seven Leaves Press.

Freud, S. (1958). The neuro-psychosis of defence. In J. Strachey (Ed. and Trans.), *The standard edition of the complete psychological works of Sigmund Freud* (Vol. 3, pp 43-68). Hogarth Press. (Original work published 1894.)

Freud, A. (1936). *The ego and the mechanisms of defense*. International Universities Press.

McCullough Vaillant, L. 91997). *Changing character: Short-term anxietyregulating psychotherapy for restructuring. defenses, affects and attachment*. Basic Books.

Neborsky, R. (2001) Davanloo's method of intensive short-term dynamic psychotherapy. In M. Solomon., R. Neborsky, L. McCullough, M. Alpert, F. Shapiro and D. Malan (Eds.), *Short-term therapy for long-term change* (pp16-53). Humana Press.

Neff, Kristin. (2011). *Self compassion*. William Morrow.

Stills, S. (1971). Change partners [Song]. On Stephen Stills 2 . Atlantic.

Ten Have-de Labije, J. (2010). *The collected writings of Josette ten Have-de Labije*. Unlocking Press.

6

SHAME IS THE GATEKEEPER

Shame creates an internal collapse that defeats healing. I view shame as the gatekeeper in therapy because doors to connection open when toxic shame leaves the body. My client beautifully described his internal experience as he recovered from a shame attack that overcame him on a lovely afternoon ocean drive. He became aware of the feelings of shame in his body and the pain they inflicted. Because he'd developed caring for his well being in therapy, he had the will to free himself from shame.

Ct: Like a thought won't even be formed in my head that I can pick up on, but my body gets totally pervaded with a negative feeling that doesn't have words. But the feeling—if I had to find words, something like, "I did something really, really wrong" or "If I weren't here, everyone would be better off without me." It's this sticky, gooey, awful feeling. That feeling, all by itself, has no words but it is a monster inside that tries to devour me. (*He is describing a non-intentional, unconscious process deriving from early memory traces.*)

Th: What a terrifying and horrible feeling!

Ct: And so if I can feel that feeling starting to sink down in me, I'm like, "I'm not going there. I haven't done anything wrong!" (*Illustrating the power of will to attend to his needs.*)

DOI: 10.4324/9780429399633-7

Th: Right, right. Wonderful!

Ct: If I'm driving along and it's a sunny day, and nothing is going on, and all of a sudden, this feeling's going to overwhelm me—what's the point of allowing that?

Th: Exactly. How terrific for you to notice this! You're describing an embodied state in which you don't feel you have the right to exist. It carries the message in your cells that you are fundamentally deficient and shouldn't be here. How far back would you say that feeling goes?

Ct: I can go straight back to being twelve and being mercilessly bullied.

Th: That's just terrible. Being humiliated is excruciatingly painful. *(He suffered humiliations much earlier in his life.)* And it's a place you can readily find yourself.

Ct: Like that!

Th: Out of the blue. Back to that whole-body state that started so young. You're suddenly feeling toward yourself an unworthiness that someone projected onto you. Degrading experiences were wired into your memory system and your body automatically goes there.

He remembers how he used to be reactive when his kids expressed negative emotions, and he'd isolate from them. He can now face his failures as a parent and feel remorse without annihilating himself. During his therapy, he unlocked the rage, grief, and love toward his parents who had also humiliated and traumatized him and set in motion a comparable pattern within himself. The client and I celebrated his freedom from the wordless, primitive shame that had invaded his body.

Shame can make a person want to disappear, die, or feel like they don't deserve to exist. Shame and fear are inextricable because shame signals that others have turned away in disgust, triggering fear that we will become an outcast and will not survive alone. Another client, Carrie, said, "Being seen is the same as being judged." Think about that. Coming into another person's field of vision is enough to set off alarms. Her raging, alcoholic mother sneered, pulled up her nose, and curled her lip in disgust when Carrie came into sight. Retracting the upper lip and mouth are "preparatory to the act of vomiting" (Darwin, 1872, p. 256). This reaction has been described as a shaming, judging face that "spits out the 'bad tasting' other" (Kaufman, 1989). Schore pointed out that disgust may be even more overlooked than shame, an affect associated with olfactory processing (Schore, 1994). Shame-based clients often perceive that others feel disgust toward them. No wonder Carrie feared eye contact, given her association that I would spit her out as her mother had done. Who would want to be seen by such contemptuous eyes! Tragically, for many clients, shame is their identity. "Why would anyone be interested in my needs and desires, my feelings or perspectives?" Such beliefs prepare the person for the abandonment they know is coming. The therapist will be no exception. In fact, therapists must struggle with their shame too!

Therapist Shame

Unsurprisingly, the more I focused on my client's shame, the more I became aware of my own. It was easy to see distancing behaviors in my clients, but shame is a two-way street. I had vulnerability around revealing my intersubjective experience and feared the client might pull away from me if I revealed my perspectives or feelings. But if I didn't take that chance, how could my clients dare to reveal themselves and how would I help them enter new places? When I failed to take necessary risks, I felt disappointed in myself.

The fear of failure and rejection inhibits both the client and the therapist. Shame is ubiquitous in therapy (Tangney & Dearing, 2011). What do you suppose is a recurring request that I receive from therapists in training with me? "Susan, could you show us some videotapes of bad sessions?" I'd shudder, but I've come to understand that therapists want to be reassured that their teachers have failures. I recently made a mess of a session with a client in crisis. I'm so grateful we could discuss what happened. I'd focused on one part of what she'd said and missed the larger picture. She felt I'd been pushing her, something I teach others not to do. But I might have avoided this injury if I had kept checking in to see how she was responding, I'm grateful that both of us took something from this experience. We forget that failure is universal. Michael Jordan said, "I've missed more than 9,000 shots in my career. I've lost almost 300 games. Twenty-six times, I've been trusted to take the game-winning shot and missed. I've failed over and over and over again in my life. And that is why I succeed." Michael reminds us that all learning requires failures to advance our skills. He should know!

Therapists feel shame when they compare themselves unfavorably to colleagues, identify with a client with similar shame issues, make mistakes in session, and experience unsuccessful treatment outcomes (Koerner et al., 2011). I find it unsettling when I see my unresolved problems show up in the person sitting across from me. The obvious question is, "How am I going to help them?" Regarding the unfavorable comparisons to colleagues, shame skews our perceptions because shame and external pressure prevents the master clinicians from disclosing their struggles and failures. To be human is to have flaws and setbacks. Be skeptical of "cures." We can take satisfaction in knowing that "the average treated client is better off than 80% of the untreated sample in most studies" (Duncan et al., 2010).

I never met a therapist who didn't question their abilities. Everyone has had clients who test the limits of our skills. Some clients stay in therapy for years, while central issues fail to budge. Clinicians watch master clinicians working and think, "I will never be able to replicate their skills. I don't have what it takes." Being a good therapist is hard. It takes considerable work, concentration, and time, and we'll need lots of compassion for ourselves. Despite periods of self-negation, discouragement, reluctance, frustration, and anger during the learning process, therapists describe a point at which the principles begin to "click" in their minds, and deep satisfaction follows. Our achievements don't mean we won't have painful setbacks. But, hopefully, feelings of hopelessness will become rarer with time. Instead of hiding our errors and shrinking from them, we could do something radically different and embrace our missteps as part of our shared humanity. What if we could feel humbled without feeling humiliated? We could use our shame to make us more relatable to our clients and more receptive to learning from them. Shame is an inevitable but temporary obstacle, not a roadblock, as we stretch ourselves in our work.

Shame is Pervasive in Therapy

Thomas J. Scheff, professor emeritus of Sociology, UCSB (University of California, Santa Barbara), said: "Shame can be considered to be the master emotion because it controls the expression and even our recognition of our other emotions, and surprisingly, of shame itself" (Scheff, 2011, p. 34). Walking into a therapist's office brings on shame. Many clients expect that their therapist will react negatively to their flaws, and they fear their therapist will also feel disgusted as they uncover unknown parts of themselves. Still, psychological healing requires unmasking in the presence of a caring, empathic other. Unattended shame will defeat therapy. "Shame settles in like a dense fog, obscuring everything else" (Morrison, 1994). We must find ways with our client's help to lift the veil of shame so a relationship can be born. We will explore the primacy of shame in treatment, how to treat shame with the Healing Triad, and we will consider the essential elements of a "shame sensitive" approach.

Is Shame a Neglected Stepchild in Therapy?

Our field has severely underestimated the clinical impact of shame work, which belongs at the forefront of psychotherapy curricula. Nathanson said that "the degree and severity of undiagnosed and untreated shame problems far exceeded anything we had ever imagined" (Nathanson, 2000). I was unprepared to handle the pervasive, nuanced, intersubjective manifestations of shame in therapy. Yet I grappled with it continually in sessions—when people's voices shrunk to a whisper, the body slumped, the eyes looked away, or vague language hid the self. Some clients manifested their shame by scrutinizing my every word, attacking me before I could attack them, and projecting their self-loathing onto me. Others telegraphed, "I'm fragile. Don't get too close. You can easily injure me. Don't intrude upon my space."

Sometimes I felt like I was touching a burn victim when working with shame-traumatized clients. I'm reminded of Heather, age 19, who told me her mother had died when she was twelve. Young male acquaintances raped her twice soon afterward. Her father was distant and disengaged. As soon as she sat down in my office, she plopped an overstuffed handbag on her lap with a pillow on top of the bag. Her arms squeezed her legs tightly together.

Th: I don't know how you've managed the pain and trauma you've endured, Heather. You lost your beloved mother and best friend at such a tender age. And then you had to cope with sexual assaults with no one to protect you. My heart aches for you.

How brave you are to come here on your own and make such an impressive effort to heal from these tragedies!

Ct: I want to make something of my life. I had straight A's before my mother died. I've been lost and depressed ever since. I want to recover the person I was. I know I have something to do in this life. But I have no energy, and I'm struggling to keep up in school. I question everything about myself.

Th: Your mother would be cheering you on for taking this brave step. I sense you have great potential to do wonderful things. But since you lost your mother and suffered two horrendous assaults, you've lost something inside yourself. Trauma has a way of shrinking us, and I think you want to take your rightful place in the world again. You must have very powerful feelings inside you, but I sense they have been deadened and now you want to come back to life. Would you agree that you must feel safe, secure, and valued, as you did with your mom, to move forward in your life?

Ct: Yes, but how?

Th: Would it be ok if we check out what your body is telling us now, about how you're feeling at this moment with me? (*Her body language telegraphed that it perceived a threat and felt ashamed.*)

Ct: I'm sitting like I always do. I don't like to leave my legs open, exposed.

Th: I'm so sad about your traumas, Heather. Deeply sad. Your suffering is heartbreaking. I think it will be important for us to talk about your painful experiences, but first, I'm concerned about your sense of safety with me. Your body is holding itself as though it perceives a threat. It's a shame for you to carry this sense of danger wherever you go. It seems like it could be paralyzing. Do you agree?

Ct: Yes, but that just how I am.

Th: I get the sense you haven't always been this way. My sense is that some mix of shame and anxiety invaded you. Does this sound right? (*She nods in agreement.*) Would you be willing to experiment with allowing your body to shift positions a bit with me, perhaps removing your bag and pillow, feeling freer to move your legs, and just see how that feels?

Ct: *I'm willing to try, but exposing my body makes me quite uncomfortable and anxious.*

> *We worked together to lower her anxiety and explore her fears. She could see she was safe in the room with me and didn't need to hold her body tightly and hide. She began to loosen. Gradually, she no longer had to hold her body as though she might be raped. We would also discover her enormous shame over her inability to function, as her mother would expect of her. My compassion became her self-compassion and dissolved much of her shame over time. In the course of her therapy, she experienced rage at her dad for his unavailability, at the men who raped her, and she eventually worked with complex feelings toward her mother. When she terminated therapy, I was in awe of the leader she became.*

People signal their shame and anxiety when they throw big jackets across their bodies, squirm and shift their hands from one armrest to the other, or sit with their arms grasping their chests or knees. We face a delicate task. We may know how to regulate affects in therapy, but how about regulating the relationship itself? Dr. Miller has said, "Of all the factors affecting outcome, the specific approach used has the smallest impact. By comparison, the relationship between client and therapist contributes eight to nine times more" (Miller, 2019). Shame is about, "Do I feel safe with you?" and "Do I feel seen by you?" I discovered that I would need to share the risk and become vulnerable with my clients to increase my attunement to them.

My clients taught me a great deal about shame, leading to a growth spurt in my skills. It was painful at times. I discovered I could perpetuate shame and not be aware of it. Certainly, the client's shame may have little to do with the therapist but there are times when it does. How often has a client told us about shame-related grievances with a former therapist, who had no idea what occurred? One client told me her therapist had treated her shame solely as an intrapsychic issue, but she was wounded that he never explored how his own responses contributed to her shame. Her reaction speaks to the client's need to impact the therapist and to be on equal footing. Maybe we neglected the cultural issues involved in the shame reaction. When we are unaware that we have activated shame, we miss opportunities to learn about ourselves and regulate the relationship. The subject of shame sometimes triggers defensiveness in therapists. It's tough to face that we've injured a client or may be uncomfortable dealing with the client's shame. If we don't find a way to talk about shame and help to separate projections from reality, we miss opportunities to deactivate shame.

A Rupture

I attempted to raise awareness of anxiety with inadequate *shame sensitivity* in the first session with Caroline. Unrepaired ruptures can pose a significant threat to treatment outcome in the early phases before a bond has formed. Injuries reenact childhood traumas: "Psychological conflict develops when central affect states of the child cannot be integrated because they evoke massive or consistent misattunement from caregivers" (Stolorow & Brandchaf, 1987). Therefore, ruptures afford opportunities to rework traumas, providing some of the most fruitful psychotherapeutic work.

Caroline came into therapy because her husband told her she had "walls." She thought that might be true and also found it hard to function after she was laid off from a high profile position in her highly successful career. The CEO, her friend Jeff, made the decision. I expressed compassion and told her about my approach, inviting her to give caring attention to her physical sensations, thoughts, and feelings as we sat together. She rapidly agreed, but I failed to explore her understanding and reaction to my suggestion. We might have avoided a rupture had I asked, "Tell me more about how this idea sits with you? It's a very new idea for most people, and I wonder how you feel about it?" Opening this discussion could reveal and normalize her reactions to embarking upon a more intimate relationship.

A vignette from this first session follows:

Th: Does that sound like something you'd want to do (giving attention to feelings, body sensations and thoughts)? That would make sense for you?

Ct: Sure, I'm open. (*I moved on too quickly*).

Th: Great! Because I'm imagining that as you're talking about Jeff and how deeply he wounded and betrayed you, you must be having a lot of feelings. As you were talking about him, you began to twist the Kleenex. I imagine this topic is difficult and may raise anxiety— (*I was hoping to raise awareness of anxiety as a response to her rising feelings toward Jeff, but Caroline cut me off before I could finish. She thought I was pointing out her anxiety as a shortcoming. I'd overlooked her shame in telling me of her humiliation and "failure," and it would have been more helpful to explore her feelings about revealing her termination to me.*)

Ct: Well, I don't know about that. It could be. In my office, I had a ton of paper clips that I played with so, it could be, but I don't relate it to umm, to anxiety. But if you say it is, I'll think about that (*her tone is clipped*).

Th: Umm, how did you feel hearing me say that? (*Thank goodness I asked that! This early lesson taught me how shaming it can feel for some clients to draw attention to anxiety.*)

Ct: Umm, I didn't understand the importance of it so—

Th: Of course, you're not in the habit of really paying attention— (*Again, she jumps in before I could finish.*)

Ct: Oh, I disagree. I think I pay attention (*indicating another injury*).

Th: —to what's going on inside of you. I'm talking about inside of you. (*I feel anxious myself, as this is going from bad to worse.*)

Ct: Because I'm playing with the tissue? (*Said confrontationally.*)

Th: I noticed you weren't fidgeting before you started talking about Jeff. (*These moments make it easy to pull back in self-doubt. But we need to hold onto ourselves and keep reaching for connection.*)

Ct: I didn't have anything in my hands to fidget with then! (*She becomes argumentative. The word "fidgeting" is poorly chosen because it has a negative connotation. One word can make a significant difference.*)

Th: But I'm just aware you weren't, you know—

Ct: I smoke too. (*She grins with sarcasm. I could see there was no way to win, and I had to deal directly with her self-protective reactions.*)

Th: Ah, huh. You mentioned that you had some walls, and I apologize for my contributions. I also sense that when I begin to pay attention to what's going on inside you, it feels like you push me away from you.

Ct: Defensive. Absolutely. I definitely felt defensive.

Th: I apologize for the way I broached this topic. I don't think I made it clear that I care a lot about your feelings. When I noticed that your hands suddenly became active at the moment you talked about Jeff, I sensed some significant feelings rising in you, and I wanted to make them important.

Ct: I see (*softening*).

Th: I also thought that you might have some unconscious fear that could make your emotions less accessible, and we would sadly miss something valuable.

She recovered from the initial injury when I could emphasize the caring behind my words. I explained that I'd linked her hand activation (a better phrase than "fidgeting") with possible unconscious anxiety related to important feelings rising. She began to get that I was trying to help her and not criticize her.

When she became less defensive, Caroline found my observation intriguing. Repairing this rupture opened the door to exploring the shame she felt in sharing her "failure" with me. She spoke of fiercely competitive feelings with women (beginning with her mother). She saw me as secure and "put together," awakening an impulse to battle for dominance. When I revealed that I was vulnerable and had limitations, her anxiety and defensiveness lifted dramatically. I was happy with the smile on her face when we ended the session. A remarkable course of therapy ensued.

Shame and Isolation Affect Health and Immune Functioning

We need others to sustain a sense of worth and integration in crisis, e.g., during a divorce or job loss. Many people minimize the universal human need to be seen, known, and valued. They will go it alone when their needs may be greatest. Evidence shows that the more extensive our social network, the more likely we are to be healthy and thriving. Several studies in psychoneuroimmunology (PNI) of the interaction between psychological processes and the nervous and immune systems show that shame causes inflammation (Dickerson et al., 2004). Increasing the capacity for healthy dependency, allowing for self/other regulation, is a central task in all psychotherapies. Shame states stymy this process.

Has Anxiety Overshadowed Shame in Psychotherapy?

Shame and anxiety are inseparable and deserve equal attention. When we reduce shame, anxiety typically drops as well. My perspective is that teachings on anxiety have overshadowed shame historically, to the detriment of our profession. Perhaps this has occurred because anxiety is a primary affect from birth that inhibits emotional expression. Some neuroscientists believe that shame comes online at twelve months, and others have said two years. Since researchers and neuroscientists differ about the origin of shame in human beings, these discrepancies raise questions about when shame affect precisely begins. I believe shame has primal roots and deserves to be deeply studied and prioritized in our work.

Are Shame and Anxiety Fraternal Twins? Can We Separate Them?

Evidence shows that shame and anxiety have overlapping symptoms, e.g., cognitive disruption, rapid heartbeat, fidgeting, and laughing over words. Studies also show the need for shame-directed approaches when shame is a source of arousal in trauma. "Anxiety and fear influence the course and maintenance of PTSD (post-traumatic stress disorder). But for survivors of IPV (intimate partner violence), there is emerging evidence of the contribution of shame to symptoms." The study continues, "A purely fear-based model of PTSD overlooks other potential sources of arousal that may affect symptoms that range from startle response to social functioning. From a treatment perspective, treating hyperarousal secondary to shame may require different approaches than treating arousal caused by fear" (Freed & D'Andrea, 2015).

Origins of Shame

I have intuitively believed that shame affect (pre-verbal, precognitive, and unconscious) is with us at birth, a precursor to feeling unworthy in relation to others, which requires later development. Shame affects are associated with powerlessness, worthlessness, unbearable aloneness, deprivation, and abandonment terror, causing protest and freeze states. The infant needs no words to experience, "my needs have no impact," and "I am alone." Failure-to-thrive babies are the most horrifying and heart-crushing examples of children deprived of touch, a loving look in the eyes, and mirroring from an attuned mother. Mary Ayers appears to view the evolution of shame similarly when she says that the infant mother's "false mirroring" results in shame:

> My theory is maternally biased, and informed by the work of Winnicott, Fordham, and Jung, whose theories are also maternally biased. It focuses on the infant's development in the first six months of life and the role that eyes play in the construction of a mother's presence and as a psychological center of their relationship. This short time frame and focus on eye-to-eye contact necessitate a close look at the mother to the exclusion of other factors. Good enough mothering and accurate reflection of the infant's needs result in strong ego development and concept of self; false mirroring results in shame. Good or poor mothering depends on the mother's level of emotional maturity; in some cases, a mother's disturbance with a particular child outweighs her capacity for love. (Ayers, 2014, p. 4)

Ayers' work suggests that shame has roots in the first six months of life, activated by looks in the mother's eyes that fail to reflect the child's experience. The infant absorbs shame from the misattuned mother, which reverberates through its later life. She presents an extensive study of the Evil Eye concept, a broadly shared belief that eyes have the power to inflict injury (Ayers, 2014). Remember my client, Carrie, who said, "Being seen is the same as being judged." In contrast, many clients have said that my eye contact communicated compassion, which impacted them profoundly. Words alone will never build a relationship.

Edward Tronick's Still Face Experiment captured the infant's disintegration and panic when the mother looked away and failed to recognize the infant's desperate attempts to evoke a response (Tronick et al., 1978). Unable to be seen by the person upon whom the child relies for survival, unbearable feelings flood the child. He collapses inwards upon himself and succumbs to primitive states of powerlessness and aloneness [states linked to shame]. A mother's unresponsiveness drives a child to shriek in protest (hyperarousal) and then freeze in despair (hypoarousal) (Bowlby 1969; Robertson, 1958). In contrast, when the mother's eyes reflect the child's value and power to impact her, he expands with a sense of safety, reassurance, and contentment. These findings provide validation that non-verbal responses can reduce shame.

Shame Starts Later

Some theorists classify shame as a self-conscious emotion, not present at birth (Lagattuta & Thompson, 2007; Lewis, 1995; Tangney & Dearing, 2002). Michael Lewis argues that self-evaluation is required to experience shame, a cognitive capacity he postulates does not occur until 18 months (Lewis, 2007). Griffin suggests that children do not experience shame until the age of seven or eight (Griffin, 1995).

Shame Starts Earlier

On the other hand, Taylor's review (Taylor, 2015) shows that "the affect of shame is not contingent on level of cognitive development" and has earlier origins than previously reported (citing Izard, Nathanson, and Tomkins). Others have described shame as a primary innate affect resulting in facial and body display (Ekman, 1972, 1973; Tompkins, 1963). "Innate" has been defined as inborn, existing from birth. "Tompkins describes negative innate affects that are present from birth and visible on the face of the newborn: distress-anguish, fear-terror, shame-humiliation, anger-rage dissmell (literally turning one's nose away from something), and disgust (similarly, turning away from something distasteful)" (Nathanson, 1987, p. 12).

While viewing oneself as unworthy or guilty requires a separate sense of self and brain maturation, feeling alone and powerless are primal. Peter Breggin, MD, tells us that guilt, shame, and anxiety are stone-age emotions that originated before the consciousness of the events that shaped them, evolving biologically over millions of years (Breggin, 2014). Guilt mobilizes us to repair the damage we have done to a relationship. Anxiety signals us that feelings need attention, but we unconsciously fear these emotions will damage a relationship. Shame alerts us that we might lose a relationship. "Shame in all its forms is relational" (De Young, 2015, p. 18). We must regulate these three "stone-age emotions" in session at all times. Otherwise, these feelings can flood the client and lead to acting out or internalization, hyper and hypoarousal. If we do not accurately identify shame, anxiety, or guilt, our attunement misses the mark. The client will not experience being "seen" accurately. The best way to get back on track is to ask the client for feedback. Clients express an unmistakable relief when our responses are on target.

The Development of Shame

The chart below (Figure 6.1) illustrates my view of the progression from the child's emotional freedom to the development of toxic shame, anxiety, guilt, and self-protective strategies. We start in life with an infinite capacity to feel, and we rely upon our parents to mirror, identify,

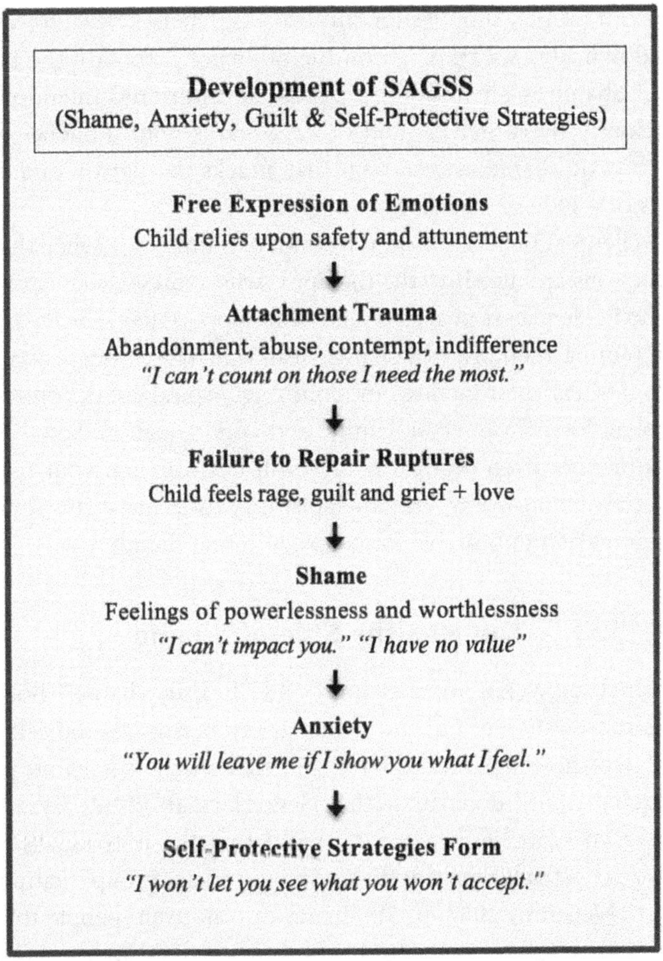

Figure 6.1 Development of SAGSS

and help manage our emotions through verbal and non-verbal cues. The imperfect though "good enough" parent will respond to the child's feelings with acceptance most of the time and help regulate the child's nervous system, providing safe outlets for emotional expression. But when the child's feelings trigger the parent's trauma, the child flounders to manage feelings they don't understand and can't regulate on their own. Thus, we become strangers to our feelings, and we develop a host of unconscious strategies or defenses to camouflage them.

"Shame is about the self, the whole self" (Lewis, 1971). Shame enters the whole body with an unconscious, nameless dread related to being cut off from human supplies for survival. As defenses develop, we learn to shut down, disappear, or go on the offensive, "You are the bad one, not me." Shame is an invader, a poison administered intentionally or unconsciously by caregivers and other humans who influence a child. I refer to toxic shame as a serpent that attacks the person and leads to paralysis or a sudden discharge of aggression.

Many clients anticipate the deep wounds of humiliation when they show their emotions and needs to the therapist, who represents an earlier caretaker who inadequately provided safety and support. Emotional expression triggers trauma memories of shame, fear, and rage, often unconscious. Many clients fear their intense emotions might spiral out of control, causing divorce, loss of career or family, and condemnation. Some imagine imprisonment or even death (my rage will kill you, and your retaliation will kill me). Some worry, "My therapist may drop me!" This shame and terror can make it unbearable for people to reveal themselves.

The Healthy Side of Shame

I distinguish between "toxic shame" and "healthy shame." Both share the emotion of shame, but the toxic variety permeates the self with a sense of worthlessness. Some have said that shame serves no purpose and is archaic, but I don't share that view. Herman (2012) says, "Shame may serve an adaptive function … regulating the individual's relation … to primary attachment figures and to the social group" (citing Izard, Gilbert, & McGuire, 2007, p. 5). Shame can motivate people to make a positive change (Lickel et al., 2014), resulting from an appropriate degree of regret for stepping outside of social bounds. Shame serves to inform us that we are too exposed, and others will not support our actions. Healthy shame can minimize the likelihood of retaliatory aggression and evoke sympathy and forgiveness (Tangney & Dearing, 2011). Shame can help us survive. A submissive, self-negating stance when encountering a gorilla, brutal king, or an abusive parent is necessary. It reduces shame to normalize it and acknowledge its survival value.

The Healing Triad: An Approach to Toxic Shame

Shame that stands in the way of therapy is toxic. As with all treatment barriers, I turn to the Healing Triad to alleviate shame:

Awareness of Shame

Therapists often try to bypass shame to alleviate their client's discomfort. We might shift from an uncomfortable topic and offer temporary relief, but we do nothing to promote change. Clients need to be aware of toxic shame and its debilitating effects to block its destructive path in their lives. Awareness includes recognizing shame's physiology (e.g., slumped posture, gaze aversion, sweating, blushing, lack of coordination, and cognitive disruption). Likewise, we note shame language: "Ridiculous, foolish, silly, idiotic, stupid, dumb, humiliated, disrespected, helpless, weak, dependent, small, trivial, uncomfortable, embarrassed, shy, vulnerable" (Herman, 2012). We also need to raise awareness of the common projections that occur with shame, highly harmful false assumptions that others view us negatively.

Therapeutic Transfer of Compassion for Self

Compassion for the suffering caused by shame ignites the will to attend to this crippling force. But where does compassion-for-self originate in psychotherapy? Typically, compassion first arises within the therapist and in successful therapy, the therapist's compassion transfers to the client. However, the shame-dominated client often believes the therapist's compassion is untrustworthy. When the client doubts and devalues us, therapists have to work harder to find compassion and tenderness within themselves. It helps to remember the trauma and suffering that created off-putting, even offensive behaviors. Sometimes we must attend to our self-regulation before we can show the compassion necessary to create receptivity in the client.

Finding Compassion within Ourselves When it's Tough

A woman sought my help because co-workers complained to her employer that she was harshly critical and they felt intimidated by her. I knew this side of her. I felt her withering disdain when she perceived that I was falling short. Though it was uncomfortable, I would need to talk with her about her contempt and how it affected our relationship.

Th: You were correct that I misspoke. After I sincerely apologized, you seemed to pull away from me, giving me the impression you would not accept my errors, which I can't entirely avoid. I feel concerned that you will focus on my flaws to the point where I will be of no use to you. We've had some powerful moments in our work together, and it feels sad should this devaluing force stop our chances at success. This makes me wonder if someone reacted to your flaws as though they were intolerable? We've seen how this shaming mechanism has taken a terrible toll on your life.

Ct: I'm glad you raised this issue and made an effort to be honest. I can see it happening.

Th: I'm so glad. What do you notice?

Ct: I know I have no tolerance for shortcomings, and my mom beat me for anything I did wrong.

The client told me about horrible childhood abuse. She sobbed. She said it felt frightening to let me get close to her, and she distrusted my caring. She also acknowledged that our relationship was sowing seeds, and she wanted to continue. Her response touched me. I could feel the warmth of compassion growing within me. Both of us took risks for this shift to occur.

Th: The suffering you've endured moves me deeply, and I appreciate your openness with me. You've been brutalized for being human. Would you want us to make it our priority to prevent this internalized abuser from doing harm to either of us? Then we'll have a chance to explore your feelings when you're disappointed in me. Does this make sense and is this a path you'd want to take with me?

Ct: I must do this if anything is to change. My answer is yes.

The Will to Embrace Feelings

When shame awareness and self-compassion are activated, the will to become free from shame typically arises. In the following vignette, the client describes how shame zaps her when she feels her power and giftedness as a public speaker. She became aware of her self-loathing and the way it shuts down her ability to think clearly. As she wrestled with her shame and released it, fury at her sister, who relentlessly humiliated her with verbal and physical attacks, rose to the surface.

Ct: After I would speak at an event, I would get the backlash from the self-hatred, but I could recognize it.

Th: Horrid feeling! And it's excellent you could recognize it.

Ct: Yeah. It's something about speaking in front of people, training them, that makes the darkness come out. Or the shame comes out.

Th: You expose yourself and then shame and judgment tell you there's something wrong with you, and it's not ok to show your power, your leadership. (*She agrees.*) This shaming force tricks you into thinking you need to be perfect, when in fact you need to be free of the shame.

Ct: Exactly.

Th: Thankfully, there are times when you're also able to see what it feels like to be free of shame when you're in a flow and connecting to others in powerful ways (*reinforcing her strengths*).

Ct: What I'm experiencing now is this pulsing, vibrating shame. It's like an electric fence. I run into the electric fence. (*Shame attacks just as I acknowledge her strengths.*)

Th: And this electric fence tries to keep you safe by telling you to shrink and hide, right?

Ct: Yeah, it's like a protection, like the judge is protecting me.

Th: Right, telling you to stay behind the fence or you're going to get electrocuted.

Ct: That kind of protection. (*Shame's purpose is survival.*)

Th: You need to stay back, not expose your unworthiness to others. (*Shame avoids the threat of humiliation and abandonment, which becomes enacted in her relationship with me.*) Tell me how it is to notice this painful shame and the effect it has on you?

Ct: Umm, I feel sad and somewhat scared, but mostly I feel this dark thing, like this vibrating shame.

Th: Umm, umm. I'm feeling a lot of empathy. That's an excruciating feeling (*hoping she will share my compassion*). What do you have to be ashamed of right now? (*Implying that she doesn't deserve her shame.*)

Ct: It feels like it's not something that I did. It's just who I am. (*She describes the invasive, engulfing quality of shame, taking over her whole self.*)

Th: Oh, I'm sitting here seeing this beautiful person—intelligent, perceptive, a deep human being who cares so much about being true and real, and who has so much to say (*countering her shame with reality*). Would you agree with that?

Ct: Yes, logically, I would. (*No feeling of caring for herself—Isolation of affect.*)

Th: I feel so sad about what's been taken from you. How does it feel to hear me say that? (*Inviting an emotional response.*)

Ct: I feel sad (*gradually, she begins to cry*).

Th: Umm. Umm. Would you be willing to stay with this painful feeling? (*Encouraging her to feel the pain caused by her shame and self-hatred.*)

Ct: And I think that I realize, like, what I'm living in.

Th: An electric fence surrounding you, ready to zap you. (*Client wipes away tears.*) It does zap you, just for existing. It doesn't give you credit. If I give you credit, I don't sound real. (*She agrees.*) Where does this sadness take you?

Ct: Um, it feels now like it just takes me down into a self-defeating place (*sadness and caring for herself turns into hopelessness*). It didn't before, but just then, it feels heavy, pressing on me. (*She's tracking internal sensations well. I attempt to refocus on her compassion for herself.*)

Th: How about if we listen to what this sadness for you is saying—if it had words to speak?

Ct: It's saying, "I'm sorry that you have to feel this way."

Th: It feels compassionate for you. (*She resists the pull toward depression. We see a moment of the Therapeutic Transfer of Compassion for Self motivating her to release the shame.*) As you recognize the pain caused by this shaming mechanism, how do you want to relate to it (*creating hope by framing shame as an entity outside her core self*)?

Ct: It's scary for me to think of not listening to it. Like I'm going to get slammed, or I'm going to get in trouble if I don't listen to it. Its voice is angry, judgmental. I notice a fiery feeling in my belly.

Th: Who makes you angry?

Ct: Well, when you said that, I see now that I think of my sister as the embodiment of that judgment. (*As shame released its grip, she processed rage toward her sister and both parents.*)

Shame Sensitive Therapy

The therapeutic growth process inevitably causes the client and therapist to question and alter themselves, evoking anxiety, fears of the unknown, and shame. Attending to shame in our clients and ourselves moves the healing process forward. We'll want to:

- Identify dysregulated shame
- Show compassion for the pain and vulnerability of shame
- Try to recognize when we unconsciously fuel shame states
- Track shame levels with our clients and ourselves just as we track anxiety

Principles of *shame sensitive* therapy:

1. Clarify if the client understands and accepts our approach
2. Seek permission to talk about shame

3 Check to see if compassion is active within us
4 Attend to our choice of words and avoid "you messages"
5 Regulate our vocal tone and inflection (prosody)
6 Examine our role in ruptures
7 Avoid the expert role to empower the client
8 Refrain from pushing the client
9 Raise shame awareness with compassion
10 Point out that an emotional treasure lies beneath shame
11 Separate the observing self from shame
12 Normalize shame
13 Bring negative projections to the client's awareness
14 Caringly attend to the therapist's shame
15 Express faith in the client's ability to surmount shame
16 Offer clear alternatives to shame
17 Risk showing vulnerability
18 Use the term "self-attack" cautiously and clarify its meaning
19 Seek to uncover complex feelings beneath shame

Clarify if the Client Understands and Accepts Our Approach

Showing a persistent interest in our client's emotions, thought processes, and bodily sensations counteracts a sense of worthlessness. We invite the client to join us in a partnership that focuses on internal experience. However, this type of intimacy often feels threatening, unfamiliar, and activates shame. The client may not be clear about the approach we propose. It's important to inquire, "Please tell me how you understand the approach I'm suggesting and how you feel about it." We don't want to proceed without permission, which means little without the client's comprehension and reflection. Does the client choose to attempt this type of intimacy with us? Pointed questions and observations can feel invasive when the client is not a full partner in the process. As we saw with Caroline, pointing out anxiety evokes shame for some people, as some cultures view anxiety as a weakness or cowardice, making people vulnerable to ridicule, humiliation, and bullying. Since anxiety is an anticipatory fear with no real and immediate danger, some fear their therapist will perceive them as out of touch with reality.

Let us talk about anxiety and other sources of suffering collaboratively, being responsive to the shame these explorations can evoke. How can we normalize, contextualize, and show caring when we discuss vulnerable states? We know it's important to discuss when a client has a pounding heart, but before asking about heart rhythms, let's seek permission first:

Th: Would you mind if we talked about what you're experiencing in your body, as this will help us help you? Our bodies know what our minds cannot. I realize that body focusing is unfamiliar to many people. Please let me know how the idea feels to you? If it makes sense for you?

Ct: It makes sense. I'm definitely not used to it. It's kinda scary. My heart is pounding pretty hard right now.

Th: I'm glad you shared that. How do you feel letting me know about your pounding heart?

Ct: It's embarrassing.

Th: I understand. Most people feel afraid of this kind of intimacy when it's unfamiliar to them (*normalizing*). Lots of feelings get stirred up in therapy. Of course, this process is very familiar to me. You said this type of sharing makes sense for you?

Ct: I see how it helps.

Th: I'm glad. Hopefully, your discomfort will become less. Do you notice any other signs of discomfort?

Ct: Just a little hand sweating. Maybe my breathing is more shallow.

Th: If you agree, I'd suggest we give attention to any of these reactions during our sessions so we can relieve you and make it possible to explore yourself more comfortably.

Seek Permission to Talk about Shame

For those who believe we need more time to build a "relationship" before we address shame, I say we form a relationship by dispelling shame sooner rather than later. Trust can shatter when we don't bring projections to light to reduce shame. How we go about this delicate task matters greatly. A "You" message like, "You look away and avoid my eyes" can feel intrusive and imply criticism, triggering defensiveness. However, we have many alternatives, such as:

Th: I noticed something shifted when you started talking about your son's difficulty getting into college, and it seemed you looked away like it's hard for you to look at me when you talk about this. I could be wrong. Would you mind if we talked about how it is for you to share with me about your son?

Ct: I feel embarrassed. My friend's kids are doing great.

Th: Yeah. I had a sense you felt embarrassed. I completely understand. I think a lot of parents feel as you do, and there is so much pressure today. I appreciate that you're letting us talk about how it is for you to let me see your pain. I'm wondering how you might expect that I'm reacting?

Ct: You might be wondering what's wrong with me. (*She allows us to explore her projections onto me and consider how her projections increase her anxiety and shame, which inhibit her ability to explore her feelings fully.*)

When therapists become more aware of the centrality of shame, they suddenly see it everywhere. "Wow, we did a lot of work on shame today!" Not surprisingly, their clients talk about their shame states more frequently as shame consciousness evolves, leading to immeasurably richer relationships.

Check to See if Compassion is Active within Us

Feelings of compassion ebb and flow within every human being. But no feeling has more impact on the therapeutic process than compassion, which needs to be directed toward both the client and the therapist throughout the process. With Caroline, I needed to remain flexible and resilient so I didn't condemn myself and potentially pull away from her. I needed to direct compassion toward myself to allow space for human error and learning. Regulating myself allowed me to communicate from a place of compassion for her need for walls and her injuries. When compassion deserts us, our clients may do the same!

Attend to Our Choice of Words and Avoid "You Messages"

This is huge. I revise my language and phraseology constantly, recognizing the impact of my choice of words on the client's receptivity to my message. Consider replacing "fidgeting" with "active hands." The former can feel more judgmental than the latter. "You are detaching" can sound more critical that "Tragically, some protective mechanism has shut down your life force." "You're anxious" vs "Your body signals a state of alarm." Some words or phrases convey more compassion than others. These subtle distinctions can have profound implications. Every exchange with a client confronts us with a choice, "What do I say and how do I say it?" Raising these questions within us carries great importance. We might revise, "You got anxious at that moment" and try instead, "I sensed your body tightened at that moment when some feelings were coming up. Emotions often make people anxious. Could we see if that might be happening with you?" Throughout the vignettes in the book, you will find commentary and illustrations of recommended language.

Regulate Our Vocal Tone and Inflection (Prosody)

My repair efforts with Caroline would have been futile if my vocal tone had not been soft and soothing. At the end of that session, she commented that I was very compassionate, and she told me she experienced that through my eyes and vocal tone. A tender tone of voice creates safety. Prosody, the lilts and drops in our voice, and our cadence all have an impact. We can develop these relational qualities with conscious intention if we recognize how we want to be with our clients and make it a part of our practice.

Male therapists have expressed their self-doubts to me about expressing softness and warmth. They question if they can practice shame-sensitive therapy. We're not going to all sound alike, look alike or say the same things, but all of us can find ways to express more tenderness and caring with conscious intention. I've been profoundly moved watching some male therapists work because I can feel the power of their loving energy and commitment. There are a multitude of ways to convey a nurturing presence.

Examine Our Role in Ruptures

When a client experiences an injury, take the time to explore how the client experiences you. A healing relationship is real and vulnerable, and everyone has defenses. Self-protective responses do not belong solely to the client. It can be more comfortable to assume that the client has projected something onto us rather than looking at how we may have contributed to a shame reaction. We may be quick to say, "It appears that I'm demeaning you, but the devaluation comes from within you." This can be a valid and helpful intervention, but there are times when the following could be more on the mark, "I can see why my response sounded sarcastic. I'm terribly sorry I came across as minimizing you." We share the vulnerability when we stop to consider our role.

When the client experiences shame triggered by real or imagined judgments or failures to read cues, anger rises toward the therapist. In response, the anger is often turned against the self or acted out with a retaliatory, demeaning statement toward the therapist. Before exploring the anger, I inquire how the client experienced me. I want to show that the client's feedback impacts me. Given that shame derives from an inability to impact significant others, nothing can be more important than providing a curative experience. When a client wants me to change something about myself, I will try to adjust my responses so long as I'm not violating my values. We do not want to replicate the expressionless mother. Shame is about powerlessness, and I want to be sure my clients know they affect me, teach me, and can change me.

Avoid the Expert Role to Empower the Client

When we make declarations, interpretations, and give instructions without collaboration, we do not support a spirit of equality and partnership. Dr. Marks-Tarlow states that "… we still get into trouble unconsciously if power motives creep to the fore unwittingly, as when we try to 'fix' our patients or change them due to our own discomforts and defensive needs" (Marks-Tarlow, 2012, p. 18). Having watched thousands of therapy hours, well-intentioned therapists become dominant frequently. "You will need to stop digressing." "Sit up." "Take the bag off your lap."

Any of us can fall into becoming directive. People frequently want to be told what to do and will pull the therapist into providing answers they would be better off finding for themselves. Being directive can feel gratifying to both therapist and client. But taking over does not build decision-making capacity and individuation, which reinforce a sense of mastery. Some collaborative responses are: "Would you be willing to give this a try?" "How do you feel about this exchange we just had?" "It's ok with me, whichever you choose." "It's so important we honor your choices here." Or "Would you want to consider allowing your feelings to move more freely through your body?" Or "How about slowing down so you can breathe more freely?" Or "How does my comment strike you?" "It looks to me like it's difficult for you to talk about your feelings toward your wife. How is it from your angle?"

I encouraged a young man to release his grief, but he held it back. He and his wife had recently lost their first child through a miscarriage, and he was terrified she wouldn't try again. I intuitively sensed that pointing out his suppression of feelings or nudging him wouldn't help. I decided to turn to him for guidance. I asked if his restraint had anything to do with me? He told me that the subtle sounds I was making distracted him. I was taken aback. No one had said that to me before, and I thanked him for his candor. As we proceeded, I stifled any vocal sounds to honor his wishes, though it felt unnatural. Silence ensued. I felt even more awkward. I was shocked when deep-throated sobs gradually broke through in waves. I sat back and appreciated his freedom to feel. I'd taken his suggestion, letting him impact me, and what a result! He became clear he had to tell his wife about his pain, fear, and desire to have another child. He was deeply relieved when she agreed to try again.

We help to build selfhood and autonomy when we relate as equals. I began a Zoom session with a couple and noticed the wife's head kept dropping below the screen. When I commented that she seemed to be pulling away, she acknowledged that she didn't want to discuss a current crisis in which her daughter had relapsed on drugs. She didn't feel like talking. Her husband continued telling his story, and I asked him what he had heard from his wife. Her message hadn't landed with him. When he could acknowledge her wish to withdraw with an accepting tone, she shared more. She didn't want advice. She'd received conflicting opinions from treatment providers about her daughter and had to rely on her instincts. I said, "When others tell you what to do, you begin to feel inadequate. You want to hear your voice." She nodded with relief. My empathy with her shame created safety, and she fully participated during the rest of the session. Her husband was happy to hear how much she valued his perspective, but she wanted him to recognize her autonomy in making decisions. When we bring internal conflicts into the open, clients can make independent choices about what they want to do. We avoid usurping decisions that belong to them.

Refrain from Pushing the Client

My client twisted in his chair as he started and stopped speaking several times. I had impulses to push him, but thankfully did not. The following exchange occurred after he'd spoken to his drug-addicted daughter, who had asked to move in with him. He found the strength and wisdom to say no but began berating himself for abandoning his children when they were young. He did something afterwards for which he was deeply ashamed. He hesitated to tell me his secret, but the choice to reveal himself belonged to him. I invited him to talk about his shame and his conflict, rather than his secret. This exchange followed:

Th: It's clearly difficult for you to tell me what happened. What do you imagine might occur if you tell me? We also might explore how you'll feel after this session ends if you don't tell me?

Ct: I think I will continue to think less of myself. I'm just beginning to enjoy feeling more of myself. I really like that.

Th: How wonderful to hear! Your sense of your value is growing, and you don't want to lose that. But it appears that shame gets stirred up about revealing something about yourself to me, and perhaps you anticipate that I will have the same bad feelings about you that you do? Does this sound right?

Ct: Yeah. It does. (*I seek validation that I've understood him.*)

Th: You expect that I'm going to view you in the same judgmental way you're viewing yourself. Would you like to tell me more about how you imagine I will react if you tell me?

Ct: I would imagine you'd be disgusted and, um, and defensive and, you know. I would imagine you'd need to put on your best poker face to, uh, to not react with disgust.

Th: You imagine that I'd be very turned off to you, very disgusted.

Ct: That's what I feel like, yeah, that you wouldn't like me anymore (*sad look*). (*In this poignant moment, I conveyed my caring.*)

Th: I feel really sad that you have such uncertainty about my acceptance of you that you imagine I would pull away from you when you are in so much pain. I also empathize with your fears about my reaction since your dad used to humiliate you horribly. This conflict is very tough for you. Let's take our time.

Ct: Yeah. Feeling this little guy in my head go, you deserve this, you are worthless. Shame on you, you rat bastard.

Th: What a cruel and nasty message you've absorbed. You've heard something similar from your dad. You assume I will react the same way. No wonder telling me feels like a tremendous risk. One part of you wants to share something to relieve your suffering, but another part fears that my response will cause even more suffering. What a painful dilemma!

Ct: Yeah.

Th: Hmm. Telling me takes a lot of courage—

Ct: It takes a lot of courage. I maybe have just enough.

He decided to tell me the source of his excruciating shame. He had urinated on himself. Seeing that I was not disgusted and did not withdraw moved him. He said quietly and with a voice full of feeling, "I know you're sad." Recognizing my caring during his agonizing self-disclosure led to profoundly deep work. We regulated his shame through my compassion for him, which allowed him to bear his painful guilt for his failures as a father. His remorse prompted him to make repairs with his adult children, without allowing them to mistreat or take advantage of him.

A colleague wondered if there are times when the therapist needs to overpower a client due to destructive behaviors. I've seen therapists bark orders, believing their passion shows caring. The client may feel at home with such responses, but dominance reinforces the one-down position. "The therapist knows more than me. I couldn't have figured this out for myself. I'm incapable of good judgment." The person suffering from shame needs more empowerment, not less.

I'm concerned when the therapist moves from a collaborator to a director, believing we can achieve the same outcome with teamwork. My tone can become emphatic at times, but I will argue against telling people what to do. We can raise challenging questions, "How will you feel sitting alone in your empty apartment when you see the agony in your children's eyes?" vs. "You're foolish to leave!" When we promote a sense of mastery, agency, autonomy, free will, and selfhood, we help to dissolve shame. Many clients are victims of humiliation. They need us to show faith in their ability to arrive at their own conclusions.

Raise Shame Awareness with Compassion

How do we use words that stir compassion and mobilize the will to release shame? Here are some possibilities:

"A monstrous shaming force attacks you mercilessly. How terrible for you!"

"Anything that attempts to destroy you is false at its core."

"There is a part of you that can observe this shaming force. How does it respond when it sees how shame is crushing your chances at happiness?"

"How tragic that you had to diminish yourself to be loved."

"What is the cost to you if this shaming force goes unchallenged?"

"A healthy part of you brought you to this office. How does this healing part wish to respond to the shame that takes you over one cliff after another?"

"I would feel great sadness if you were to allow this diminishing bully to control your life."

Point Out that an Emotional Treasure Lies Beneath Shame

Let clients know that shame blankets their vital feelings with tragic consequences, and that their emotions are a rich treasure and necessary to their well-being. Use any examples to bring this reality to life. Help the client to see the self-protective, archaic and detrimental function of shame. They may have needed to become small when faced with a parent who would hit them or scream at them, but those days are over. They no longer have to hold their head down, muffle their words, bow their shoulders, and bury their feelings. They can separate from shame if it is their will, thereby clearing a path for their feelings to break through and breathe freedom.

Separate the Observing Self from Shame

We help our clients to see that they are not their shame and have the option to separate from it. The therapist might say:

> "You're able to observe your shame in action, and you want liberation from it. Your awareness and desire are parts of you that are different from your shame. An unhealthy force has wrapped its vines around your core, but the vines are not you. Shame can prevent access to your emotions only if it's given that power. You were born with the capacity to feel. It is your birthright. You had no choice as a child but today you have the ability to release your shame and experience your feelings. And I'll be right there supporting you."
>
> Another illustration:
>
> "It looked as though a dark force invaded you, making you appear smaller than you are, causing you to doubt yourself. Do you sense this is happening, too? (*Listen to see if the words resonate.*) Do you agree that there's a part of you that lives outside your shame, that can step back and see what this toxic shame inflicts on you?" (*With sufficient self-compassion and will, the client can cease being at the mercy of the serpent of shame.*)

Normalize Shame

Let clients know that they absorbed shame from others through no fault of their own. Any child is at the mercy of their parents and can be poisoned by shame. "Who would not feel shame and humiliation when you were relentlessly criticized?" Help the client to see that they are not to blame for their shame, and shame does not belong to them. Universalize shame. Everyone knows the pain and shame of rejection by people who matter. "Adopting the viewpoint that shame is a normal state which accompanies the breaking of affectional bonds allows shame to take its place as a universal, normal human state of being" (Lewis, 1981). When therapists reveal their own struggles with shame, we help to normalize and universalize this most human emotion. We might say, "I too have been subjected to bullying and remember the agony of those experiences well."

Bring Negative Projections to the Client's Awareness

When we discuss our clients' doubts and distrust of us, we pave the way to connection. When we inquire, "I wonder how you imagine I'm seeing you or reacting to you at this moment?" The client may respond:

"You looked disapproving."

"Will you like me or want to work with me if you see the real me?"

"If you discover how afraid I am, will you view me as a coward or see me as weak?"

"Will you be disgusted by the intensity of my needs?"

"Will you tell me I'm abnormal or think I'm insane (*dread of the diagnosis*)?"

Anyone with a childhood caregiver who was depressed, hostile, chronically overwhelmed, ill, or self-absorbed will hide dependency needs. We hide what the parents rejected, so they could accept the rest of us. What could affect the therapeutic relationship more profoundly than the belief that our therapist judges us? If projections are operating, clarify the client's direct experience of the therapist. "Do you see anything that suggests that I'm judging you?" "Could we explore what you're noticing about me?" Rather than argue (a dead end), we can be curious and draw out what the client experiences to begin a mutual self-reflection process. In dealing with projections, I like to share my experience with the client to establish a sense of reality. "I feel quite fond of you" or "I was feeling a lot of compassion for you at that moment." If the client can see that I am not judging, I will then explore the feelings that accompanied the projection. "If it were true that I was disgusted with you, you must have feelings toward me. Could we explore those feelings?"

Caringly Attend to Our Own Shame

How do we respond to ourselves when we recognize our shortcomings? Perhaps we have transmitted judgment or distaste, or we feel impatient or angry with a client. Therapists can do harm, and shame can prevent us from honest self-reflection. One of my most cherished writers, Anais Nin, described her analyst's questions as "thrusts," as though she had suffered an inquisition. She felt oppressed, dominated, and dismissed and this exchange took place:

> Anais: Today I frankly hate you. I am against you.
>
> Dr. A: But why?
>
> Anais: I feel you have taken away from me the little confidence I did have. I feel humiliated to have confessed to you. I have rarely confessed. (Nin, 1966, pp 85-86)

"Not infrequently, reports from therapists explain away failures by means of labels attached to patients, which, however fashionably couched in technical terms, can be roughly translated, 'It's all your fault.'" (Meares & Hobson,1977). We may feel ashamed, but can we own our flawed humanity with compassion? Therapists can be excessively harsh judges of themselves, but isn't it far better to be curious instead? A therapist who had scored above the upper limits of performance in Dr. Scott Miller's sizable research project (Miller, 2007) described how she responded to a woman who showed the slightest negative facial expression during a session. The therapist entreated her client to share the meaning of her microexpression, and the client dodged her questions. But the therapist persisted in a kind and curious way. The woman eventually disclosed that the therapist had a look on her face that conveyed disapproval to her. The therapist asked the client to replicate the expression, and the client made a particular face.

The therapist then recreated that same expression and asked her client if she got it right. She had. Then she went to her husband and showed him the facial expression and asked if he recognized it? What courage! He responded that he'd seen it many times and didn't find it favorable. The therapist began to practice replacing that expression with something more inviting. This therapist's willingness to examine how she contributed to a shame response is impressive. Her *willingness to actively practice new behaviors* contributed to her exceptional performance. Our faces telegraph unconscious messages all the time, and it's admirable to check to see how others perceive us. This type of exchange with our clients helps to determine what originates from within them and what belongs to us.

Express Faith in the Client's Ability to Surmount Shame

A woman left my office after a moving course of therapy and said, "It was your faith in me that made the greatest difference." Shame is about not being seen and valued. Faith recognizes the capacity and the potential in the client and makes it real. However, drawing attention to strengths means little if the client doesn't recognize them too. For example:

Th: I'm impressed you fought back when your shame tried to silence you. Do you see your improvement too?

Ct: Maybe.

Th: Seems like you're hesitant to join me in acknowledging you, and I wonder how is it to have both of us recognize your progress?

Ct: I was told not to draw attention to myself.

Th: Shall we take a look and see how this serves you?

Offer Clear Alternatives to Shame

"Would you be willing to replace your shame with self-caring by dismissing the devaluing voice inside you?"

"Would you consider turning away from those old familiar judgments and just notice what feelings emerge?"

"Precious feelings lie underneath your shame at this moment. If you reach for them, they will speak to you, but only with a genuine invitation. You'll discover that your feelings are some of your best friends."

Risk Showing Vulnerability

Do as we teach. Sometimes letting our guard down gives our clients hope by showing them what it is to be free of toxic shame. Admitting our errors without whipping ourselves or collapsing is a great model for our clients. Daring to be authentic helps dissolve shame.

Th: You're not alone with this. I had a terrible struggle to let myself feel anger too.

Ct: Really? I wouldn't have imagined that. You seem so confident. I don't feel so bad.

Th: You only see a part of me. I'm vulnerable too.

Use the Term "Self-Attack" Cautiously When Discussing Shame

Many dynamic therapies treat shame as a defense and a form of self-attack. I believe this orientation has implications for practice and theory. Some analysts have described self-attack as an unconscious process that enacts past relational traumatic memories in which we've learned to dismiss, negate, neglect, and loathe ourselves.

However, most clients and therapists hear the term "self-attack" as something we're doing to ourselves. While "self-attack" or references to self-harm raise awareness that we have choices that carry consequences, the language we use to describe internalized punitive forces can create unintended shame. The idea of "self-attack" leads to interventions like, "You avoid declaring yourself." Or "You dismiss yourself again." When I've mentioned self-attack with clients, they've often told me, "Now I have something else to feel ashamed about." An attacker is associated with abusiveness and evil. Therefore, people often see an attacker as a shameful part of themselves. I seek to use language and concepts that evokes compassion, helping people become aware of toxic operations within themselves that are primarily unconscious, learned, automatic, self-protective, and stemming from childhood. I want my clients to know that self-harming behaviors and responses alert us to trauma and victimization. For example:

Ct: I don't believe I've accomplished anything.

Th: I feel the tragedy of your beliefs. I sit before a woman of such depth, wisdom and creative spirit who has impacted the lives of countless people, family members, and mine as well. Yet, you've breathed toxins from your early environment, and the messages you've absorbed into yourself negate truth and reality about who you are. I wish I could just lift this burden from you that sucks the life from your creative potential. But I can do nothing without you. I believe in us. Will you care for you as I care for you, so we can triumph over all that negates and diminishes you, so your voice can be heard and appreciated at last?

Seek to Uncover Complex Feelings Beneath Shame

When we cover ourselves with a blanket of shame, we become impotent. In this state, we're unlikely to ask, "How do I feel about the person who humiliated me?" Perhaps we said something foolish, impulsive, or we weren't thinking. We sent an errant email; we stood up a friend; we got the date wrong for a meeting; we made a poor choice of words, or we were insensitive to someone's needs. Maybe we didn't do any of those things, but someone is annoyed, and we don't know why. The person we offended ghosts us, or erupts with fury, or degrades us in front of others.

Shame-prone people absorb these devaluations or lash out, cutting off the opportunity to explore all of their feelings. A man looked at me with lifeless eyes and asked, "What is the point of feeling my anger?" I answered, "What is the point of feeling love and grief and joy?" He became quiet and reflective. "Emotions give us life!" he said. "Is there a point to feeling alive?" I asked. He answered his own question, and his will to feel came online. He allowed himself to feel the heat of his rage, which morphed into intense love for his wife. Another man described his mother as a "Medusa," with multiple snakeheads who bit chunks out of his identity. Who would not feel paralyzed when confronted with such a monster? But surely anyone would have instincts to remove the head of the Medusa. When the client did just that, she could also connect to her deep compassion and love for her mother, who had suffered unspeakable traumas. When we regain the right to feel all of our impulses to destroy, grieve, and love, shame dissolves.

Pete could not have healed without access to his complex feelings. He was terrified I would "see" his rage. Shame triggered a temporary paralysis. We will see how shame often commingles with fear. Pete felt boiling rage toward his violent father (Warshow, 2002). When I invited him to explore his feelings with me, he suddenly jumped up from his chair.

Ct: I can't express it. I feel weird (*throws his arms out in a gesture of powerlessness and shame*).

Th: Why?

Ct: I feel weird throwing my hands out, or uh— (*Swings his arms again. "Feeling weird" suggests shame. Being seen is new and unfamiliar.*)

Th: Would you mind coming back to your chair and allow us to talk about the energies you're experiencing in your body, Pete? Your feelings were never encouraged before, so talking about them feels unnatural and shameful.

Ct: Yeah, I don't want you close to my anger.

Th: You want to protect me, yet we abandon your anger. That's sad! You don't want us to get close to vital emotions within you. Yet, how do we give you the help you need if we banish your feelings? I say this with great empathy because I know you've had experiences that make it terrifying to expose what you feel.

Ct: This reminds me of Stan at work. (*He diversifies with a story about someone else, a protective strategy.*)

Th: If we talk about Stan right now, I sense it will take us further from your vital anger.

Ct: You're probably right, but I want to avoid it.

Th: I hear you. I get it. You want to distance yourself from your feelings, and of course, you can. I've no doubt this habit was necessary early in your life, but you are in a new time and place. You said your wife left you because she said she couldn't know you. If you move away from your anger, might this habit of shutting down continue with me?

He fidgets and looks away while anxiety and shame rise together. He faces a hard conflict. If his feelings remain hidden, he cuts himself off from relationships. But if he exposes what he feels, he believes something catastrophic could happen.

Th: You look very uncomfortable in your body, Pete. Could we talk about what you're noticing in your body?

Ct: My heart's pounding. I can feel it down to my hands. I feel tense.

Th: Thanks for telling me. Tell me more about your tension. (*He raises his shoulders.*)

Ct: I don't know. I feel stiff as a board.

Th: Your whole body?

Ct: Yeah.

Th: So, your anxiety spiked terribly and does it seem hard to look at me?

Ct: Uh huh.

Th: How distressing for you to be at the mercy of these forces that shut you down at the thought of letting me get closer to you and this anger. How would you describe the price you pay for avoiding your feelings?

Ct: (*Pause*). Live a life that sucks.

Th: In what way does it suck, Pete? Would you tell me more? (*Exploring the cost of self-protective habits often ignites the will to feel.*)

Ct: Oh, uh, not feeling good about myself. You know, not being happy to be me.

Th: Yeah, a punishing force slams you into silence and self-contempt.

Ct: Screwing with my head.

Th: Yes (*pause*). What do you think is the effect on your relationships with other people?

Ct: I think it keeps me at a distance from them.

Th: That's such an important insight. Could we say this is happening with us? I'm not saying we don't care for each other, but something prevents you from letting me know you fully.

Ct: That's true.

Th: What do you feel when you think about the price you pay? *(Ideas without emotion will not bring change.)*

Ct: Um, just pretty lonely. I don't have, uh. I don't have, uh, real closeness in my life—with anybody.

Th: That is tragically true, Pete. I wish we could make it otherwise.

Facing the reality that his distancing habits impact our relationship and my ability to help him stirred a state shift. He saw the necessity of transparency. Pete took the monumental risk of telling me that he had fantasized about how he would kill his violent father as an adolescent and had never told anyone. For the first time, he processed intense fury toward both parents. I felt privileged to be part of such a meaningful moment of freedom in his life. He experienced that he could have his feelings and not be banished by me. He told me later that a day in his life hadn't gone by when he didn't think of his father with hatred. The next session revealed this had begun to change.

Ct: I feel like I made enormous progress with my feelings about my father and came to a place of acceptance, forgiveness, and serenity that I've never had before. I realize that I love my Dad. (*He was able to recover a memory of a toy his dad had carved for him. I was joyful to learn that Pete had happily married a terrific woman post-termination and was depression-free eight years later.*)

When Pete could distinguish between feelings and actions, he saw that his rage did not harm, and he became freer. Realizing that his fury was a protest against being attacked and humiliated by his father, he became more compassionate toward himself. He saw that he'd only wanted to be loved by his father and he began to feel empathy for him too.

People often confuse losing control of emotions with the human right to feel. I sometimes ask people, "If we explore your anger, do you imagine you'd tear my office apart?" Usually, the person grins with relief, knowing this won't happen. Allowing our feelings to course through our veins and our muscles liberates us. As self-other affect regulation develops in the therapeutic relationship, the client can safely choose the time, place, and manner of healthy emotional expression.

References

Ayers, M. Y. (2014). *Mother-infant attachment and psychoanalysis.* Routledge.

Bowlby, J. (1969). *Attachment and loss.* Basic Books.

Breggin, P. R. (2014). *Guilt, shame, and anxiety: Understanding and overcoming negative emotions.* Prometheus.

Darwin, C. R. (1872). *The expression of the emotions in man and animals.* John Murray.

De Young, P. (2015). *Understanding and treating chronic shame: A relational/neurobiological approach.* Routledge.

Dickerson, S. S., Kemeny, M. E., Aziz, N., Kim, K. H., & Fahey, J. L. (2004). Immunological effects of induced shame and guilt. *Psychosomatic Medicine, 66*(1), 124–131. https://doi.org/10.1097/01.psy.0000097338.75454.29

Duncan, B. L., Miller, S. D., Wampold, B. E., & Hubble, M. A. (2010). *The heart & soul of change: Delivering what works in therapy* (2nd ed.). American Psychological Association.

Ekman, P. (1972). Universals and cultural differences in facial expressions of emotion. In J. Cole (Ed.), *Nebraska symposium on motivation, 1971* (Vol. 19, pp. 207–282). University of Nebraska Press.

Ekman, P. (1973). Cross-cultural studies of emotion. In P. Ekman (Ed.), *Darwin and facial expression: A century of research in review* (pp. 169–222). Academic Press.

Freed, S., & D'Andrea, W. (2015). Autonomic arousal and emotion in victims of interpersonal violence: Shame proneness but not anxiety predicts vagal tone. *Journal of Trauma & Dissociation: The Official Journal of the International Society for the Study of Dissociation (ISSD)*, 16(4), 367–383. https://doi.org/10.1080/15299732.2015.1004771

Griffin, S. (1995). A cognitive-developmental analysis of pride, shame, and embarrassment in middle childhood. In J. P. Tangney & K. W. Fischer (Eds.), *Self-conscious emotions: The psychology of shame, guilt, embarrassment, and pride* (pp. 219–236). Guilford.

Herman, J. L. (2012). Shattered shame states and their repair. In J. Yellin & K. White (Eds.), *John Bowlby memorial conference monograph. Shattered States: disorganised attachment and its repair* (pp. 157–170). Karnac Books.

Kaufman, G. (1989). *The psychology of shame: Theory and treatment of shame-based syndromes*. Springer.

Koerner, K., Tsai, M., & Simpson, E. (2011). Treating shame: A functional analytic approach. In R. L. Dearing & J. P. Tangney (Eds.), *Shame in the therapy hour* (1st ed., pp 91–114). American Psychological Association.

Lagattuta, K. H., & Thompson, R. A. (2007). The development of self-conscious emotions: Cognitive processes and social influences. In J. L. Tracy, R. W. Robins & J. P. Tangney (Eds.), *The self-conscious emotions: Theory and research* (pp. 91–113). Guilford.

Lewis, H. B. (1971). *Shame and guilt in neurosis*. International Universities Press.

Lewis, H. B. (1981). Shame and guilt in human nature. In S. Tuttman, C. Kaye & M. Zimmerman (Eds.), *Object and self: A developmental approach* (pp. 235–265). International Universities Press.

Lewis, M. (1995). Embarrassment: The emotion of self-exposure and evaluation. In J. P. Tangney & K. W. Fischer (Eds.), *Self-conscious emotions: The psychology of shame, guilt, embarrassment, and pride* (pp. 198–218). Guilford.

Lewis, M. (2007). Self-conscious emotions: Embarrassment, pride, shame, and guilt. In M. Lewis, & J. M. Haviland-Jones (Eds.), *Handbook of emotions* (2nd ed., pp. 623–636). Guilford.

Lickel, B., Kushlev, K., Savalei, V., Matta, S., & Schmader, T. (2014). Shame and the motivation to change the self. *Emotion*, *14*(6), 1049–1061. https://doi.org/10.1037/a0038235

Marks-Tarlow, T. (2012). *Norton series on interpersonal neurobiology. Clinical intuition in psychotherapy: The neurobiology of embodied response.* W Norton & Co.

Meares, R.A., & Hobson, R.F. (1977). The persecutory therapist. *British Journal of medical psychology*, 50, 349–359.

Miller, S.D. & Hubble, M.A. (2011). The road to mastery. *The Psychotherapy Networker*, *35*(2), 22–31, 60.

Miller, S.D., Hubble, M.A., & Duncan, B.L. (November/December, 2007). Supershrinks: Learning from the field's most effective practitioners. *The Psychotherapy Networker*, *31*(6), 26–35, 56.

Miller, S. D. (2019, December, 22). Where did you get that idea? *scottdmiller.com*. https://www.scottdmiller.com/where-did-you-get-that-idea/

Morrison, A. (1994). The breadth and boundaries of a self-psychological immersion in shame a one-and-a-half-person perspective. *Psychoanalytic Dialogues*, 4(1), 19–35. https://doi.org/10.1080/10481889409539003

Nathanson, D. L. (1987). *The many faces of shame*. Guilford Publications.

Nathanson, D. L. (2000, March 18). A Conversation with Donald Nathanson (G. Levin). Behavior Online. https://behavior.net/2000/03/a-conversation-with-donald-nathanson/

Nin, A. (1966). *The Diary of Anais Nin*, vol. 11. Swallow Press and Harcourt, Brace & World (Harvest Book).

Robertson, J. (1958). *Young children in hospitals*. Basic Books.

Scheff, T. J. (2011). Shame as the master emotion: Examples from popular songs. In J. G. Lacey, R. Jewett, & W. Alloway (Eds.), *The shame factor: How shame shapes society* (pp. 30–39). Cascade Books.

Schore, A. N. (1994). *Affect regulation and the origin of the self*. Erlbaum.

Stolorow, R. D., & Brandchaft, B. (1987). Developmental failure and psychic conflict. *Psychoanalytic Psychology*, 4(3), 241–253. https://doi.org/10.1037/h0079136

Tangney, J. P., & Dearing, R. L. (2002). *Shame and guilt*. Guilford Press.

Tangney, J. P., & Dearing, R. L. (2011). *Shame in the therapy hour* (1st ed.). American Psychological Association.

Taylor, T. F. (2015). The influence of shame on posttrauma disorders: Have we failed to see the obvious? *European Journal of Psychotraumatology, 6*, Article 28847.

Tompkins, S. S. (1963). *Affect, imagery, consciousness: II. The negative affects.* Springer.

Tronick, E., Als, H., Adamson, L., Wise, S., & Brazelton, T. B. (1978). The infant's response to entrapment between contradictory messages in face-to-face interaction. *Journal of the American Academy of Child Psychiatry, 17*(1), 1–13.

Warshow, S. (2002). Treatment of a self-defiling, recovering alcoholic with an avoidant personality. *AD HOC Bulletin of Short-Term Dynamic Psychotherapy, 6*(1).

7

ANXIETY

Static on the Airwaves

Relational security is the most penetrating of all relaxants, the sense that we will be seen, heard, felt, and held by another. If we felt secure in our relationships with others and ourselves, we would be far less likely to feel anxious. Our clients seek a state of safety with their therapist, but their formative experiences tell them that their feelings will damage relationships. Many people who seek therapy are unaware of their need for emotional connection, but we find a vulnerability and even terror of rejection beneath their facades. Fear mobilizes the animal's body to protect itself physically (Panksepp, 1998), and anxiety mobilizes us to defend ourselves psychologically (Freud, 1926). Freud also believed that people feared that their drives would be punished (1923), and Davanloo theorized that unconscious complex feelings and impulses drove anxiety (Davanloo, 1995). Anxiety has also been associated with anticipatory fears as differentiated from fears due to immediate and real threats.

From my perspective, some anxieties can involve conflicts over feelings and some may not. Many people feel anxious that others will punish or victimize them for their ideas, beliefs, feelings, racial identity, gender identity, past behavior, family secrets, socio-economic background,

DOI: 10.4324/9780429399633-8

and other personal identifications. This kind of anxiety may not always involve a fear of feelings, an intrapsychic conflict, or a need to erect toxic types of psychological defenses. I believe that staying open to the sources for anxiety in particular circumstances refines our attunement. All anticipatory fears may go back to a fear of pain, but not all pain involves psychological conflict or defenses.

Existential anxiety also has a major impact on psychological health. In some cases, we can do no more than empathize or we might work with a habit of destructive rumination. Giving attention to anxiety in all its forms becomes crucial to being able to participate fully in life and pursue our dreams and vital interests.

Anxiety Builds When Neglected

Many clients have unnamed fears and body dysregulation that they routinely ignore, which heightens their anxiety states. A young, depressed, obese woman with diabetes continually twisted and pulled her hair, a signal of anxiety. Her projections onto me, driven by self-hatred, increased her sense of threat. We had agreed we would notice her bodily signals and feelings.

Th: Would you like us to notice what you're experiencing in your body?

Ct: I hate any attention to my body. I'd prefer to focus on the thoughts in my head. To be honest, the suggestion makes me mad.

Th: Thanks for telling me. Of course, we won't do anything you don't want to do. You mentioned you gave a lot of attention to your thoughts in your prior therapies. Do you believe if we do more of the same, it will help you?

Ct: (*Her eyes enlarged.*) Probably not! Nothing has worked.

Th: What if the "answers" you seek will involve more than your mind?

Ct: That's a revolutionary idea! (*She pulled up her slumped body and looked directly into my eyes.*) I fear you will give up on me and see me as hopeless as my other therapists have.

She revealed her abandonment fears and projection onto me, giving us essential insight into her relentless anxiety and hair twisting. She had no faith that change was possible and never thought her body signals would provide a way forward.

Th: I will not give up on you. Who is it that feels hopeless? I hurt for you when you say you hate giving attention to your body. I sense an intense, shaming, and rejecting force that's living inside you, and it starts looking like the rejection is coming from me. You fear that I will leave, but don't we see a part of you that gives up on you? And I'm aware of the part of you that brought you here has courage, and wants something new.

Ct: I do feel hopeless about myself and hate that I feel hopeless. (*She begins to weep.*)

Th: Perhaps it's good that you hate the hopelessness that underestimates you.

Ct.: I never pay attention to anything good that I accomplish.

Th: Do you want to change that with my help? If so, we need to give attention to all of you, including your body and feelings. (*Her perception that I had no faith in her changed by the end of the session.*)

Most of us would frantically try to get a clear signal if we heard an emergency alert on the radio. When anxiety alarms go off, such as shortness of breath or brain fog, many ignore this "static on the airwaves." A better option is to work with the dial to decipher the message. Some stop listening to the radio altogether to avoid the whole unpleasant experience. We forget to ask, "Why am I having this reaction at this particular time? What triggered it?" Our clients need help to recognize anxiety reactions as vital cues to underlying feelings, and they haven't discovered that anxiety will lift when feelings are free. Anxiety will not release its grip without attention. We can't help a client attend to anxiety if the client doesn't see it, name it, or care about it. When we draw attention to anxiety, with shame sensitivity, we express compassion and move closer to uncovering the trauma that drove the anxiety in the first place.

Assessing Anxiety Levels

The more severe the anxiety, the more attention it requires. Our anxiety assessment tells us when it is safe to shift gears and move toward underlying feelings. If we underestimate anxiety and fail to sufficiently regulate it, we can set off regressive or repressive states and heighten ANS (autonomic nervous system) dysregulation (See Figure 7.1).

Sympathetic Nervous System	Parasympathetic Nervous System
• Dry mouth • Dry eyes • Dilated pupils • Increased sweating • Cold hands and feet (blood is shunted to the large muscles in the arms and legs) • Gastrointestinal tract (decreased motility) • Bladder (constricted sphincter) • Increased heart rate, blood pressure, and respiration • Shivering • Piloerection (muscles contract) • Hands cold and sweaty • Blushing	• Salivation • Teary eyes • Constricted pupils • Migraines • Warm hands • Gastrointestinal tract (increased motility: nausea, vomiting, diarrhea) • Bladder (relaxed sphincter, urge to urinate) • Decreased heart rate, blood pressure, and respiration • Dizziness • Foggy thinking • Bodily anesthesia • Limpness

Figure 7.1 Symptoms of Sympathetic and Parasympathetic Nervous System Dysregulation

Frank Anderson has written:

> ... most extreme reactions resulting from trauma fall under one of two categories: sympathetic hyperarousal and parasympathetic blunting. Understanding what happens in the nervous system when clients experience sympathetic activation (a state of high physical energy, high emotion, and low ability to regulate and calm things) and parasympathetic blunting, or hypoarousal (characterized by low physical energy, low emotion, and low access to cognitive functioning), orient me ... when confronted with trauma symptoms in the therapy room.
>
> (Anderson, 2016)

In high hyper or hypo-arousal states, a client could hyperventilate, suffer a migraine, irregular heart rhythm, or diarrhea. One of my clients had a history of going to the ER due to fainting episodes triggered by panic attacks. In one session, after sharing negative feelings toward a friend and positive feelings toward me related to his progress, he began to have a severe anxiety reaction:

Ct: You've been a huge help. An enormous help.

Th: Well, we're a good team.

Ct: I have a relationship with you like I've never had with anyone. I've had several attempts at therapy in the past and never felt a relationship like this. Totally different. I never got to the bottom of things like this, the real side of things. I never got there. (*He begins to look down and holds his head with one hand. He looks away, and I sense him disconnecting.*)

Th: Are you looking at something?

Ct: No, I'm sorry. I'm feeling a little bit dizzy.

Th: You are? (*I feel concerned given his history of fainting. He says, "Yeah."*) Really? Don't say you're sorry. I'm so glad you told me. Tell me more.

Ct: It just happened. Just like that.

Th: Do you notice anything else? (*Encouraging his observing self to speak to me.*)

Ct: Some kind of very peculiar, distant feeling. It's the kind of feeling I used to have before I would faint. (*I felt alarmed.*) I think it's emotional.

Th: Your anxiety really shot up. Anxiety can cause fainting. (*He says, "I know."*) Well, I don't want you fainting. (*This is said with a bit of emphatic humor to relieve tension. We both laugh, and he lightens.*)

Ct: I'll try not to. Talking about it helps. Being able to talk about it, it helps. (*This is very valuable for therapists to remember: Talking and reflecting helps reduce anxiety.*)

He became regulated fairly quickly by identifying his symptoms, and our relationship reassured him. He was able to have strong breakthroughs to complex feelings after this episode without high anxiety. In a follow-up four years following his termination, he told me his fainting episodes had never recurred.

Another client vignette illustrates attention to high anxiety and shame work:

Th: I'm so glad you told me about getting diarrhea after you saw your ex-husband. How is it to share that with me (*realizing that diarrhea is a common source of shame*)?

Ct: Quite embarrassing.

Th: I thought it might be, as it's difficult for most of us to discuss. Yet it's so helpful you brought it to our attention. How do you imagine I might react?

Ct: It's a pretty disgusting topic.

Th: We can all relate to this experience. This symptom tells me about your suffering, and by telling me, you help me to help you. (*Vocal tone matters.*) It looks like anxiety triggered your diarrhea, as there are no medical explanations, and your symptoms appear alongside high emotion. It's so important we give immediate attention when your anxiety gets high. How do you feel hearing this?

Ct: Better about talking about it. There's a sort of relief. I think you're right that this is more likely to occur when I'm upset.

Th: I'm so glad you feel relief talking to me and see a link between your diarrhea and a rise in feelings. Your body doesn't feel free to feel and begins to shut down. If we create safety around your feelings through our relationship, you'll be able to feel without shutting down. Do you have any urges right now?

Ct: No. My stomach was churning a bit, but it isn't anymore. I like what you're saying. It gives me hope I won't have to live with this hideous symptom.

Th: Would you be willing to tell me anytime you have stomach disturbance in the future? And to talk about any other signs of anxiety that I may not be aware of?

Ct: I'll try.

Th: It will be so crucial to our ability to help you. Your embarrassment, a type of shame, makes you suffer alone. What do you say to the two of us making sure that you're not alone? (*She agreed.*)

I dropped the charged subject of her ex-husband and her feelings toward him quickly because her high anxiety symptoms required immediate attention. A general rule of thumb: Detour immediately from highly charged feelings, impulses, and material that sets off anxiety at approximating a level of 7–10 on a scale of 1–10. See Figure 7.2 for high anxiety symptoms of smooth muscle discharge and cognitive disruption. Striated muscle discharge typically indicates a tolerable level of anxiety, but we have to assess the amount of discomfort it causes. Exceptions can occur. The client who told me that his whole body was "stiff as a board" had entered a type of freeze state, and his anxiety clearly needed regulation. Employ anxiety regulating methods,

Pathways of Anxiety Discharge	
Striated Muscle Pathway of Anxiety Discharge	• Thumbs and hands (clenched) • Arms, shoulders, neck (tense) • Head (tension headache) • Chest (intercostal tension, sighing, hyperventilation) • Abdominal muscles (tension) • Feet and legs (tension)
Smooth Muscle Pathway of Anxiety Discharge	• Bladder (urgency, frequency) • Gastrointestinal (spasms, IBS) • Vascular (migraine, hypertension) • Bronchi (Asthma) • Legs (weakness, "jelly legs") • Gut (Conversion, the client looks relaxed)
Cognitive/Perceptual Pathway of Anxiety Discharge	• Drifting, dissociation, going blank, losing track of thoughts, loss of receptive, and/or productive language, poor memory • Blurred vision • Ringing in the ears • Dysfunction/loss of other senses • Hallucinations • Fainting and dizziness

Figure 7.2 Pathways of Anxiety Discharge.

such as those described below, until anxiety lowers to a tolerable level. The therapist and client team will need to carefully track changing bodily sensations to not miss significant fear states. Many symptoms of anxiety cannot be recognized until the client tells us, which requires a degree of safety and self-caring.

The subjective experience of mid-range anxiety (5, 6 on a scale of 1–10) is not as concerning and typically takes less time to reduce. Anxiety below level 4 can often be moved past rapidly, with a few comments. This subjective assessment of anxiety relies on observable phenomena and the best intuition of both therapist and client. I will often ask the client to help us identify the scale of anxiety and physiological distress.

A male client was prone to dissociating and developing asthma symptoms when anxious. especially when he approached his anger. As his tolerance for feelings increased, he progressed to having tightness in his chest and mild shallow breathing when feelings rose. Bringing his rage and guilt to consciousness with compassion lowered his anxiety. In a regulated state, he became able to identify fury toward an old friend, who was unreliable and non-reciprocal, as a "tornado" in his core. As his therapy continued, his asthma symptoms markedly lessened.

Sometimes therapists overestimate anxiety and underestimate the client's capacity to bear feelings. We may hyper-focus on anxiety and continue to "regulate" it after anxiety has reached the "window of tolerance" (Siegel, 1999). The therapy hour runs out, and the opportunities to reach fertile emotions pass. It is usually safe to proceed with emotional exploration when anxiety manifests as mild to moderate muscle tension (see Figure 7.2 Striated Muscle Pathway). An example of manageable anxiety would be, "I feel a tight band around my stomach" or "I feel my hands clenching."

Sample intervention for striated muscle activation, in which we encourage feelings to surface:

> *Th:* What a shame that your muscles squeeze and restrict the flow of your emotional energy, robbing you of the freedom to feel. Would you want to invite your feelings to move out of your chest and through your body? Where do they want to travel?

Therapists Have Anxiety Too

Therapists hesitate to delve into feelings because of their fears of the unknown. "Can I handle intense emotions, and what will I do with them?" I caution therapists not to berate themselves when they are cautious. I held back many times before I dove into deeper emotional territory. Devaluing ourselves makes us more avoidant or overly eager, and we're more likely to miss vital signals. With time, study, and practice, we can learn to recognize the physiological signs of hyper and hypoarousal and be ready to co-regulate them.

Therapeutic Tools to Diminish Anxiety

1 Reduce shame related to anxiety
2 Explain why it's essential to share body sensations

3 Show compassion for the suffering caused by anxiety
4 Demonstrate expertise in working with anxiety
5 Advocate for the client's freedom from anxiety
6 Normalize anxiety by clarifying its context and universality
7 Monitor the client's will to attend to anxiety
8 Raise awareness of bodily signals with *shame sensitivity*
9 Share your observations about anxiety with permission
10 Avoid focusing on emotions when anxiety is high
11 Work collaboratively to diminish anxiety
12 Unravel distorted perceptions and other defenses that raise anxiety
13 Highlight current capacities not available in childhood
14 Reinforce that the relationship is safe
15 Separate anxiety from co-mingled feelings
16 Awaken compassion for the suffering caused by anxiety
17 Draw causative links between anxiety, feelings, and defenses
18 Use tender vocal tones, facial expressions, and embodied engagement

Reduce Shame Related to Anxiety

Anxiety inhibits emotional expression, and we need our client's help to identify and regulate it. People often feel ashamed of their anxiety, making them less likely to disclose it. Some fear their anxiety makes them appear irrational or weak. We can normalize anxiety by commenting that it is universal and place it within the context of early trauma. "Someone taught you to fear exposing your feelings." Here's an exchange to reduce shame over anxiety:

Th: I empathize that it can feel embarrassing to tell me your heart is pounding. Most of us are reluctant to expose uncomfortable physical sensations. I appreciate your openness because it helps us so much to be able to help you. As you allow me to know what's going on in your body, how do you imagine I'm reacting to you? (*Getting negative projections into the open.*)

Ct: I don't feel like you're judging me,

Th: That's great because I'm not. I also notice that judgment comes to your mind.

Ct: Yeah. I often feel judged.

Th: Maybe you unconsciously fear that I will also disapprove.

When therapists point out anxiety in blunt and seemingly unfeeling ways, we can create more shame. Although the therapist may have compassion, it does little if the client can't feel it. When it looks like someone is feeling nothing, they're likely to be unconsciously anxious. As we compassionately draw attention to unconscious defenses like detachment, anxiety rises to the surface along with shame. We can then help to regulate these states.

Explain Why it's Essential to Share Bodily Sensations

If we remain unaware of anxiety levels in therapy, concerning symptoms can increase, like migraines, irritable bowel, or nausea. My greatest fear as a therapist was to cause harm. Learning to work well with anxiety on the road to emotional exploration has given me far more confidence, although success requires two active partners. It is up to me to be sure my client knows what that teamwork entails as we go along, should the client choose to work with me.

An example of an active alliance:

Th: John, it seems like you lost track of your thoughts, which can happen to any of us when we become anxious. Were you aware of feeling anxious right now? Do you notice anything going on in your body?

Ct: I feel queasy.

Th: Thanks so much for telling me. These reactions tell us your anxiety shot up, which is very stressful for your body. It will be vital for our work to let me know about these sensations, as it's the only way we can help you break free from your distressing anxiety.

Show Compassion for the Suffering Caused by Anxiety

Th: I'm truly sad that you get these terrible anxiety headaches, especially when your mom comes over. Anxiety causes you so much suffering. It feels awful in our bodies and we see how it can affect our health. It's held you back from having what you want and being able to enjoy it once you get it. If we work together in a very focused way, paying special attention to your anxiety, I think we'll succeed, and you'll find more freedom for your feelings.

Demonstrate Expertise in Working with Anxiety

Our clients will not trust us with their anxiety if they don't see us as competent.

> *Th:* It helps a lot that you let me know your legs became weak. We sometimes call this jelly legs and it's a sign of fairly high anxiety, which happens when very intense emotions get triggered in you. We've also seen your shallow breathing and sudden stomach cramps when feelings run high. Fortunately, we have several ways to regulate these anxiety responses so you can be freer emotionally (*telegraphing that the path to healing is emotional freedom unhindered by anxiety*). We'll both have to give immediate attention to these symptoms if we are to impact them.

Advocate for the Client's Freedom from Anxiety

An advocate means business. It's someone who won't desert you and will even fight to set things right. Anyone who's been hospitalized knows what it means to have an advocate. They're worth their weight in gold, I want to advocate for the client's freedom from anxiety.

> *Th:* I will stand firmly for your right to have your emotions without repression and stomach spasms. I hate for you to be functioning below your capability in your career and to be unable to enjoy your new baby. These are terrible losses. With your permission, I will help you keep an eye on your anxiety, understand the triggers for it, and experience how we can regulate it together. If it's your will to give attention to your anxiety, we can make a difference as a team.

Normalize Anxiety by Clarifying its Context and Universality

Our clients need to feel they're not deficient because of anxiety. An example follows:

> *Th:* When you risk exposing your emotions, your anxiety spikes. I imagine someone has terrified you for showing your feelings, and this may have occurred at a young age. Many people have this experience, and our body remembers everything. However, more secure relationship experiences can rewire the brain, and what happened in the past can be left in the past. Hopefully, our relationship and a connection to your feelings will give you the safety you need to heal.

Monitor the Client's Will to Attend to Anxiety

As I've said, desire is the engine of treatment. Desire motivates us to grapple with the obstacles that stand in the way of our goals. Anxiety is one of the barriers (SAGSS) that poison the quality of life and stunt our dreams. Anxiety recedes through vigilant, active engagement on the part of both client and therapist. Progress relies on partnership, period. A client may learn to identify anxiety and share observations with the therapist but still do nothing toward self-regulation. Disengagement must be brought to the client's attention, not to scold but to inform that suffering lurks without the client's involvement. We have a duty to inform, not control. A sample intervention:

> *Th:* You've courageously declared your will to express your feelings without anxiety. So much is at stake in the years ahead. We can ask, "Will your marriage be satisfying, will your career flourish, will you enjoy your kids?" It's wonderful how you've grown in your ability to recognize your anxiety, but a passivity or helplessness prevents you from intervening in your suffering. Your meditation classes and exercise routines stopped (which helps your anxiety), and there's a habit of looking the other way when rumination takes hold of you. I've seen you bring your anxiety down, which we call self-regulation. I'm with you all the way, but nothing will get better without your engagement.

Raise Awareness of Bodily Signals with Shame Sensitivity

Unless we identify anxiety, how do we most effectively work with it? We can treat anxiety in implicit, relational ways or by using a variety of techniques, but how does the client recreate this process outside of our office? I prefer right and left brain integration when working with anxiety, combining the experiential with explicit understanding. If we call attention to anxiety without *shame sensitivity*, the client will be more likely to block our efforts (see Caroline, Chapter 6).

Central to attunement in psychotherapy is assessing low, moderate, or high states of anxiety. Invite the client to share any bodily sensations invisible to the eye so that the therapeutic partners can work together to provide relief quickly. It takes two to lower anxiety, and while the therapist can facilitate a powerful healing connection, we can do nothing lasting and deeply curative alone.

As I attempted to raise one man's awareness of anxiety, the following exchange took place. He described himself as a "bully," and he internalized highly combustible rage. He had persistent suicidal ideation lasting several years. We began with a discussion of body signals:

Th: Do you want to see how it feels inside your body right now as we're talking… any feelings or sensations like muscle tension or other physiological signals?

Ct: Yeah, my shoulders are very tense and rising upwards. I was holding my breath and can almost feel pain in my chest. It's like I can't take a breath, and I get very fidgety.

Th: It's so helpful that you can observe your sensations. (*Reinforcement of cooperation is important.*) I'm noticing your shoulders tightening. How is it feeling to talk to me about this distress in your body, which suggests anxiety? I know it's new to reveal yourself.

Ct: Yeah, it's very weird. It's difficult. I never talk about how I'm feeling. (*He habitually hides from others.*)

Th: Yes, I know (*said with sadness in my voice*). It's new for most people, and you're not alone. Opening up can feel extremely risky (*normalizing his shame and anxiety*). As you said, you feel most comfortable "under the covers." I imagine it's a huge step to come here and open up to me.

Ct: Yeah. You're right. I do have a lot of anxiety.

Th: Your body tells us you don't feel safe. Danger signals go off. Right?

Ct: Yes. My breathing constricts. (*If a client should begin to hyperventilate, my voice intuitively becomes tender. Steady vocal tones, speaking slowly and caringly, soothes fear states. The very act of engaging the client to reflect collaboratively eases anxiety.*)

Th: Thanks so much for telling me about your physiological reactions. We sure don't want you to have difficulty breathing! I sense that it feels unsafe to just be here with me. Seems like this shortness of breath comes up around revealing yourself to me? (*Clarifying the source of his fear helps to de-escalate it.*) I suggest we just stay in this present moment between us. Do you know that I'm here with you? (*Reinforcing the attachment relationship.*) Can you tell me more about what you're experiencing with me?"

Ct: Yes. I don't talk about myself. Never. (*He validates that I understood correctly, and he takes a long exhale.*) I don't get close to people.

He discloses his distancing defenses. We proceed with valuable shame work, and he visibly relaxes. His breathing becomes steadier.

Share your Observations about Anxiety with Permission

I often urge therapists to share their perspectives, whether related to anxiety or other internal phenomena, after receiving a general permission to do so. This point may appear obvious, but many therapists keep their valuable observations to themselves! Why? Therapists may fear the client's reaction or minimize the value of their insight. When this happens, both therapy partners lose a lot.

This client was anxious after telling me about his progress in therapy. He was rarely satisfied with himself, and he feared I would judge him for bragging. This negative projection stirred complex feelings toward me, which he repressed. His anxiety and self-condemnation caused him to pull at his cuticles. I would learn he frequently caused his cuticles to bleed.

Th: You were saying you notice a difference from last week?

Ct: Yeah. (*His hands fidget significantly.*)

Th: What do you see is different from last week? And is it ok if we keep our eye on anxiety? (*He agrees.*) Because I'm noticing there's a lot of energy in your hands, right?

Ct: Yes.

Th: Do you associate that with anxiety? Or tension? What's your sense of what that is? (*Inviting collaboration.*)

Ct: I think it's not so much anxiety but a self-soothing thing. I know people who pinch their nails. Somebody pointed out that I do that too.

Th: Well, let's consider that when we are soothing ourselves, our bodies are experiencing a threat, and we're attempting to calm our fears. Does that make sense? (*Creating the space for the client to integrate a new idea.*)

Ct: Yes. I hadn't seen it like that before.

Th: Right. If you felt safe right now, you wouldn't need to soothe yourself.

Ct: Yeah.

Th: What does it feel like to just leave your hands at your side?

Ct: OK. But if I stop thinking about not moving them, they're going to go back.

Th: I suggest you become aware that fidgeting reinforces anxiety and does nothing to lessen it. Instead, we could look at why you became anxious as you told me of your progress. (*He remembered his dad had "whacked him" when he showed pride, and his projection onto me triggered his anxiety and repression of his feelings.*)

In the following example, the client was argumentative when the therapist shared a perspective. Therapists can feel distressed when their observations fall on deaf ears. Perhaps the client rejects or ridicules us, and the therapist may retreat in silence. But when we disappear, little of real value will occur. When the client is dismissive, acknowledge this fact without judgment and resist trying to change anything:

Th: I'm noticing that you pull back when our perspectives are different. You have every right to disagree, and everything I say won't be on target for you. I also know you're seeking some new perspectives on what's going on within you that is outside of your awareness, and I'm wondering how that happens if you don't choose to consider my ideas for you?

Sometimes therapists feel pressured to catch every body signal, and anxiety causes them to sound robotic or non-relational. "You just tightened your hand, and your body twisted in your chair. Now your leg has a kicking motion." Our best comments are organic and not jarring or humiliating. When we speak with compassion and invite collaboration, an alliance is more likely to form. We don't have to mention every instance someone fidgets or smiles over a feeling, but a comment will help when pronounced fidgeting or incongruous smiling impedes closeness.

Avoid Focusing on Emotions When Anxiety is High

Move away from feelings immediately and toward anxiety regulation when a client hyperventilates, gets nauseous, loses train of thought, or has other symptoms of significant ANS dysregulation. Most importantly, we can calm fear states by raising awareness that the client is not alone. Be sure the client knows you care and are with them. Eye contact, empathy, and attunement are paramount. For example:

> *Th:* Wow, this topic triggered a lot of feelings and anxiety, didn't it? Let's take it slowly and just notice the process that unfolded here, and know that I'm with you, and you're not alone. Do you know that? (*Wait for eye contact and recognition of the relationship.*) It looks like your strong emotions about your dad overwhelmed you and caused you to lose your train of thought. This cognitive disruption seems a lot like what happens in your committee meetings when the manager gets nasty. Does it make sense to you that you become afraid of your strong feelings, and then you can't think? (*If yes, "Tell me how it makes sense to you."*)

Encourage the client to talk aloud and reflect together. A series of interpretations can raise anxiety higher because the material may be hard to process. However, a simple overview can help. Go slowly, engage, make eye contact, and help the client feel the safety of your relationship. Some sample responses:

> *"Do you know I'm with you and that you're no longer alone?"*
>
> *"You're here with me now. Your trauma is in the past."*
>
> *"Tell me how you understand what just happened within you."*
>
> *"It seemed you got anxious around your feelings toward your dad. Does this make sense to you?"*

We can shift from the right-brain to the left-brain, becoming cognitive, and utilizing the observing ego to reflect on what started the dysregulation. Therapists can use their clinical intuition to select an effective anxiety-reducing technique (Levine, 2008; Ogden, 2006; Shapiro, 2001). Anxiety regulation can occur in less time than many therapists expect. Once anxiety is lowered, we can safely return to a graded approach to the exploration of feelings. In this case, we'd do better to start with feelings toward the manager than the father, because the feelings won't be so overwhelming toward a current figure (Malan, 1979). We'll want to check frequently to assess anxiety levels.

Work Collaboratively to Diminish Anxiety

To impact anxiety levels, we can't go it alone. Help the client to become clear about their role in helping us to help them. We don't want to create the impression we have powers that don't exist.

The client's role in reducing anxiety:

1. Noticing and sharing anxiety feelings in the body with the therapist
2. Recognizing the cost of anxiety
3. Reflecting on triggers for anxiety (causality)
4. Choosing to absorb the therapist's compassion for suffering due to anxiety
5. Taking the risk of allowing closeness with the therapist
6. Grieving for the suffering caused by anxiety
7. Experiencing complex feelings on the other side of anxiety
8. Working through early traumas and separating the past from the present
9. Refocusing. We can't give full attention to two things at the same time. When anxious, the client can refocus on a project, go somewhere that soothes and relaxes (the beach, a garden), read a book, meditate, walk, exercise, track body sensations, refuse to accept anxiety-provoking thoughts, or talk to a friend.
10. Eating healthy foods
11. Choosing reciprocal, secure, loving relationships
12. Reinforcing hope and challenging ideas of despair
13. Engaging the will to leave anxiety behind

A collaborative process unfolded when a woman entered my office seeming a bit disoriented and distracted. She cognitively disrupted in our conversation, alerting me to high anxiety. I helped her to recognize her anxious state and asked, "Do you have a sense of what is driving your fear?" Without my question, she wouldn't have volunteered to tell me that a man who camps outside our building had become aggressive more than once with her. She disclosed that she still felt fear from these incidents, and we discussed the misfortune that she would have endured her fear alone if I hadn't shown interest. She revealed that she didn't want me "to feel bad" or see her as "a complainer." She anticipated my judgment and recognized this projection was due to her sense of unworthiness.

I helped her to see that I felt compassion for her fear and sense of aloneness. After the session, I contacted our building management asking for additional protection for my clients, and the man moved on. When my client knew I'd made an effort for her, she felt more hopeful and empowered. She directly experienced the value of voicing her feelings and needs.

Unravel Projections and Other Defenses that Raise Anxiety

One client had repetitive experiences of being "disrespected" by others. This traumatic theme had plagued her since childhood, and she found "disrespect" in most of her relationships. She became alarmed and angry when this happened, but quickly minimized her anger, believing it to be an unattractive emotion. When she complained of her boyfriend's "disrespect" for not removing some trash from her trunk, as she had requested, I suspected projection and splitting. She had described him as very considerate of her in the past, so he demonstrated he valued her. She agreed that neither of us could say with any certainty that he had no respect for her. The truth is that she has little respect for herself.

She pushed back on my initial attempts to raise her awareness of projection and splitting by diving into other stories about her boyfriend to make her case. I saw that arguing would be futile and suggested we could each have our points of view. I left some silence around my words. I then shared my belief that her assumptions could do her a lot of harm. When she sensed my caring and became interested in my perspective, I reminded her of the profound sense of deficiency nestled inside her. She often believed others saw her the way she did. I said that she and her boyfriend were different people, and he'd undoubtedly been leaving trash in his car for much longer than he'd known her.

Once she recognized her projection, she expressed enormous relief from anxiety and could laugh at her certainty about his motivation. A light bulb went off, and she said she wished she'd seen this 20 years ago. She went on to recall other relationships in which her projections and splitting sabotaged her. These defenses were a significant source of her anxiety. I added that I saw a need to undo the shame over her rage. She had suffered many cruel humiliations in her formative years and needed a place to process her rage. She built the capacity to allow her rage in therapy.

The following exchange is another example of defusing a projection that activated anxiety:

Th: When you revealed you had intense anger toward your sister, your body jumped (*almost imperceptibly*), as though you were in real danger for showing this emotion. Did you feel that?

Ct: Yes. I don't like talking about anger. I kinda left the room. (*Dissociation.*)

Th: Exactly. So glad you're aware. Your anxiety really spiked. How about if we explore the source of the danger? Since there are only two of us present, how might you be harmed for expressing your anger?

Ct: You wouldn't find me attractive.

Th: Let's check in with your real experience. I know you have anger toward your sister. Would you mind taking a look into my eyes and tell me if you see any signs that I'm reacting negatively to you? (*Her direct experience is more useful than an explanation.*)

Ct: No. You look very accepting of me. It's me who doesn't accept myself. (*Her recognition of her projection lowered her dysregulated state immediately, showing the power of examining the defenses.*)

Let's imagine the client had responded, "Yes. You looked uncomfortable when I said, 'I'm angry at my sister.'" While she might be projecting, she might also have picked up something unconscious in me. It's best to explore. "Can you tell me what gives you this impression?" Maybe I'd looked away, intellectualized, or showed a flash of anxiety or disapproval in my eyes. These things happen. If this occurred, I'd want to acknowledge the truth apologetically, without self-devaluation. There is a way to feel regret without diminishing ourselves: "Thank you for bringing this up, and I did move away from your anger, which is certainly not helpful. I'm committed to staying with your emotions and to working on myself too. I'm sorry I left you at that moment. How is it to hear me say this?" (*Not until the rupture heals would I inquire, "Could we return to looking at how you felt this anger toward your sister? I am truly interested."*)

Anxiety and defense trigger one another. Feeling alone increases anxiety, which triggers defenses, which creates more isolation and more anxiety. Decreasing anxiety and reducing the need for self-protective strategies allow people to feel closer and therefore less anxious. The anxiety that is related to exposing feelings underlies almost every distancing mechanism that we encounter.

Highlight Current Capacities not Available in Childhood

Th: Your trauma was then. It's in your rearview mirror. Now we're here. Powerlessness is in the past.

Th: You no longer require my approval, and I am a different person from your mother.

Th: Can we come back to the safety we've experienced together?

Reinforce that the Relationship is Safe

"Do you sense that I am here with you now?" This simple question can radically reduce feelings of aloneness. When we check to see if the client senses our support, we lay the first bricks to build a bridge. I asked this question of a woman who was in a downward spiral of regressive fear. My eyes and my words seemed to hold her as she gained a foothold:

Th: You are identifying right now with what that little kid felt. But who is it that's able to look at this little girl's experience?

Ct: Me.

Th: You. And are you a little kid now? Aren't we two competent women?

Ct: Yes (*said through tears*).

Th: Do we not have a lot of life experience? And we don't have to be intimidated by anybody. Do you agree?

Ct: I agree.

Th: This is a memory of what this frightened little girl went through, and how overpowering your mother was, and how brutal she was. But you would agree, we don't have to be afraid.

Ct: No. It's just very traumatic when I think about it. It's just sad.

Th: Yeah. I'm sure you have a lot of feelings. You were sad and angry that she would dominate, brutalize, and terrorize you. Do you think we might just look at those feelings from where you are today, this strong woman you are who does not need to be intimidated by your mother? A woman who has a friend in me.

Separate Anxiety from Co-mingled Feelings

A woman described how a fellow student directed a racial slur at her when she was in her late teens. She said she felt like beating this person up, a rare disclosure as she had strong resistance to her impulses. As we explored her fury, she began to get a headache, neck tension, dry mouth, and stomach upset. She also felt ashamed of her passivity. She was terrified of her rage and strongly associated anger with violence, which had frequently erupted among her family members. Her anxiety had repeatedly stopped us from going further in our sessions, and I decided to take a leap, "If you didn't become afraid or ashamed, might we look at how this anger feels like releasing from your body?" She surprised me by imagining pummeling the student with her fists to the point of "semi-consciousness." She felt the activation in her hands. She described a new sense of empowerment afterward. Here we had separated her angry impulses from her anxiety, a start toward setting her feelings free.

Awaken Compassion for the Suffering Caused by Anxiety

Th: I call anxiety "static on the airwaves." A pure emotional signal tries to reach you, but bringing your feelings into the open scares you, and your stomach turns over. The movements of your feelings are like waves that turn back on you and make you nauseous. These waves want to reach the shore.

Ct: Interesting. I do get motion sickness on boats. Now you're talking about motion that comes from within.

Th: Exactly. You experience tightness in your throat and chest, like "an elephant sitting on you." What do you feel about this monster trying to crush you?

Ct: I don't like it.

Th: That's great! It's terrible that a thief robs you of the freedom to feel. I hope you'll tackle this monster and allow me to help you. I'll stand next to you if you want to open a path for your feelings to enter.

Draw Causative Links between Anxiety, Feelings, and Defenses

When we help clients recognize that emotions can trigger anxiety and self-protective mechanisms due to a lack of perceived safety in relationships (Davanloo 2000, Malan 1995, Abbass 2015), we have identified a cause and and implied a solution to the person's suffering. The client may wonder, "Maybe I don't have to be afraid of my feelings or believe every fantasy in my head. Maybe my assumptions about this person are wrong, and I'm safer in this relationship than I thought. I could take a chance to be who I am." As one client responded, "I don't want to go through life afraid of my emotions."

I'd mentioned a client who often had asthma attacks when she was intensely angry. When she could see that her anger triggered high anxiety leading to asthma symptoms, instant repression and detachment, she became curious about her anxiety over anger. She realized that she feared she might become violent, like other family members, and could possibly harm someone. Putting this together opened amazing doors to exploring her emotions without shortness of breath or cognitive disruption.

A man with ADHD was in a panic during a couples session:

Th: When your wife shows displeasure, you have strong feelings that arise rapidly and are outside your awareness. Your feelings trigger a panic reaction and then your mind makes assumptions that she will leave you because of your ADHD. Let's see what we can do to lower your anxiety so you can tune in to your own feelings and also hear what she's actually saying. (*After regulating his anxiety, he could hear his wife's reassurances and became aware of the power of his projections to terrorize him. He had a big Aha! moment.*)

Ct: Wow! That's really true. I'm getting afraid of things I make up in my head.

Th: Yes!! And this is a horribly painful habit. Would you want us to tackle it together?

Use Tender Vocal Tones, Facial Expressions, and Embodied Engagement

A scholar in the field of nonverbal behavior, Albert Mehrabian, considers vocal tone, intonation, and volume to account for 38% of communication, and he attributes as much as 55% to body language, describing it as "more important in interpersonal relationships than language itself" (Mehrabian, 1981). Ekman and Friesen (1969) term the non-verbal dimension the "relationship language." The prosody of our words and phrases have an impact, making our comments more or less likely to land in the unconscious subterranean layers.

Some words and phrases are imagistic, memorable, multi-dimensional, and lush in their ability to invite creativity and move emotions. Words can connect or estrange. Just one word or phrase might sever a relationship or make it sing. Attending to vulnerable states of anxiety calls for *shame sensitivity*, compassion, and an awareness of the power of words.

Allan Abbass, MD, tells us that hearing the therapist talking can bring down anxiety. For this to happen, I imagine the therapist's vocal tone is regulated, kind, and reassuring. The steady voice itself can be a reminder that all is well. Talking together and hearing our voices as we make meaning together appears to have an anxiety-reducing effect. When the therapist can make sense of disturbing phenomena, anxiety drops. Clients with extreme anxiety have said that focusing on my voice or face enabled them to calm themselves. Being silent can make anxiety go higher. While silence can be powerful at particular moments, silence causes some people to feel alone and abandoned. Projections thrive in silence. Respond to the clients' disclosures with words, sounds, expressions and body language that implicitly communicate, "I am here."

Relationship is the Antidote to Anxiety

As I think about my most satisfying therapeutic experiences, those clients demonstrated a willingness to enter into a profound relationship with me and with themselves. I can use every skill I possess, but nothing is possible in therapy without the client's ultimate decision to take the high dive and allow closeness between two people, the therapeutic partners. A psychiatrist who had found relief from his chronic anxiety with both

CBT (Cognitive Behavioral Therapy) and intensive dynamic therapy had relapses. He knew how to regulate his anxiety, but he didn't practice the methods that worked for him. He disengaged from himself, and reverted to the belief that his anxiety was biochemical. For long-term positive outcomes, this client needed a long-term, caring, reliable relationship with himself as well as with others. Will we value ourselves enough to show interest in what triggered our anxiety and invest energy to relieve it? Attention to anxiety doesn't mean endless self-absorption, but it does mean a willingness to care enough for ourselves to engage with our anxiety.

Rachel sat across from me with her head dropping downwards into her hand, her open fingers covering her face, her thick curls tumbling forward into the space between us. I yearned to relieve her pain and was ready to welcome with compassion any feelings or thoughts she wished to share. However, she said she "had no energy for the work" of relating today. Her charismatic lover had left her at the insistence of his wife. She sought my help because she wanted relief from a long, painful pattern of powerlessness and loneliness. She also wished to "know herself." Yet her fears stood in her way. She worried she would be less desirable to her boyfriend if she became empowered. That possibility existed, but how could anything good come from an impoverished relationship with herself? In the world she knew, she had to crush her feelings to survive.

She feared her emotions would turn her into an out-of-control, demanding shrew who sobs and screams hysterically. In fact, she had hurled insults at her boyfriend when he left her, and she blamed her outburst for his withdrawal. I agreed that cathartic outbursts were very harmful, but her intense emotions deserved a safe place where they could be recognized and explored. Rachel had no experience of sharing and metabolizing feelings without the co-mingling of dysregulated anxiety and shame. Both of these toxic affects would need to decrease for healthy, adaptive affects to have a space to exist. I would need Rachel's help to reduce her anxiety and shame.

However, Rachel's belief that her boyfriend, like her mother, would prefer a submissive slave drove her to grasp her fantasies tightly at any cost. For Rachel, taking her internal experience seriously was the same as stepping into an abyss. Experience told her that self-engagement would lead to abandonment. Two defined people could not co-exist in a relationship. Later I learned that she liked living separately from her boyfriend, where they could come and go and never have to encounter the messy sides of each other and disappoint one another. Sleepless nights and depression had exhausted her, but she declined my recommendation for a medication evaluation.

The mere act of looking at me, seeing compassion in my eyes, and my invitation to give attention to her internal experience, brought on high anxiety, moments of dissociation, and then sudden collapse. She did not allow us to attend to her anxiety. I was sad and noticed some anxiety in myself when she asked to end the session early. She created distance between us, as she did in all her relationships.

The decision to stop early was hers, and she reacted gratefully when I accepted her desire to withdraw. It was rare in my practice for someone to end a session prematurely. In the next session, she told me about other relationships in which she'd suddenly shut down in a similar way. She'd recently cut off a friend, saying she "felt overwhelmed" and "had to get out of there." She provided an opening to approach what had happened between us.

Th: You are saying that your sudden withdrawal from your friend was much like what happened with us last time. I think you became anxious when I asked how you felt in your body, as you talked about your boyfriend. Abruptly, a curtain descended. You needed to leave and be alone. Does this seem right? (*My observations would mean little without collaboration.*)

Ct: Yes. It's the same. I get overwhelmed, and I have to go.

Th: It's very sad to me that you feel you must be alone at those moments of distress and strong emotions.

Ct: What else could I do? (*Her poignant question touched me. I wanted to convey my compassion for her sense of terrible aloneness.*)

Th: I'm very saddened that it's foreign to you to seek help when you're hurting. I know you don't know me, but It seems that in your inner world, you do not see others as a source of safety and support. This aloneness has been excruciating for you. I know you contacted me to discover something new. I'm here for one reason only, which is helping you. You've said that you need stable relationships, and that's a wise voice within you. Rather than draw conclusions about people without evidence, you might turn toward your friend and let her know of your distress. You could ask for her help in understanding what happened between you. (*Suggesting she check out her frightening projections.*)

Ct: I would feel very exposed. That would be very different for me. (*She took a long exhale.*)

Th: Yes, I know. It would be entirely new to share that you have needs and feelings. You would be vulnerable, but there might be room to repair your injury and hers. When you asked to stop the session with me, you had become overwhelmed. It seems such a shame that you go it alone. Perhaps you could turn to me, so we might discover what triggered your sudden fatigue. We might find a way to just be with your feelings without having to pull away from me.

Ct: You ask me questions, and I can't know the answers.

She reveals an important clue. Clients often perceive the therapist's questions as a quiz, expecting the teacher to pounce on a mistake. When I asked about her feelings toward her boyfriend, the man she loved and needed, fear instantly repressed her rage and complex feelings. Shame also silenced her as she thought she couldn't meet the expectations she'd projected onto me.

Th: I'm so glad you mentioned a problem with my questions. Honestly, I don't seek "answers." I have no expectations of you at all. I never want to ask questions without your permission, and it's so important that we can clarify your wishes. You said that you wanted me to help you know yourself and "find your center" (*referencing her desires for therapy*). My questions invite an internal discovery process. Tuning into your body is like sitting with a friend, quietly noticing what arises. I'm wondering how we get to know you more deeply if we don't show any interest in what goes on inside you, so you won't have to suffer alone?

Ct: That would feel better. I don't know how to do it, but I don't like the way I can't face anything.

Th: I think that's great that you want something better for yourself than leaving yourself. To do this, we'll need to notice what's going on in your body, any sensations that might occur. It looks to me like you become anxious right before you check out. Anxiety grows when we ignore it, and it's so sad to neglect your body's distress signals and do nothing to assist you (*Therapeutic Transfer of Compassion for Self*).

Fortunately, Rachel did become curious about her anxiety and internal experience, and her will to engage in therapy began.

People feel astonished to learn that the relational trauma they most fear has already occurred. Only extreme circumstances would make us as powerless and utterly dependent as we once were as children. We are no longer trapped, and we do not have to accept abuse, neglect, or indifference to our feelings, either from others or ourselves. As adults, we have far more options for dealing with our emotions and getting our needs met. Many people are significantly surprised to learn that the most significant relationship threat they face today stems from how they interact with themselves!

References

Anderson, F. (2016). Responding to extreme trauma symptoms: How neuroscience can help. [Blog post]. www.psychotherapynetworker.org/magazine/article/1056/in-consultation

Davanloo, H. (1995). Intensive short-term psychotherapy with highly resistant patients. I. Handling resistance. In H. Davanloo (Ed.), *Unlocking the unconscious: Selected papers of Habib Davanloo* (pp. 1–27). Wiley.

Ekman, P., & Friesen, W. V. (1969). The repertoire or nonverbal behavior: Categories, origins, usage, and coding. *Semiotica*, 1, 49–98.

Freud, S. (1959). Inhibitions, symptoms and anxiety. In J. Strachey (Ed. & Trans.), *The standard edition of the complete psychological works of Sigmund Freud* (Vol. 20, pp. 77–172). Hogarth Press. (Original work published 1926.)

Freud, S. (1961). The ego and the id. In J. Strachey (Ed. & Trans.), *The standard edition of the complete psychological works of Sigmund Freud* (Vol. 19, pp. 3–66). W.W. Norton. (Original work published 1923.)

Levine, P. (2008). *Healing Trauma*. Sounds True.

Malan, D. H. (1979). *Individual Psychotherapy in the Science of Psychodynamics*, Butterworth.

Mehrabian, A. (1981). *Silent messages: Implicit communication of emotions and attitudes*. Wadsworth.

Ogden, P., Minton, K., and Pain, C. *Trauma and the body: a sensorimotor approach to psychotherapy*. W.W. Norton.

Panksepp, J. (1998). *Affective neuroscience: The foundation of human and animal emotions*. Oxford: Oxford University Press.

Shapiro, F. (2001). *EMDR*. (2nd edition). Guilford Press.

Siegel, D. (1999). *The developing mind*. The Guilford Press.

8

GRAPPLING WITH GUILT

When someone we love is suffering, we suffer too. A mother said to her son, "Your pain is my pain." Guilt requires empathy, the ability to enter into the experience of the other. A husband said to his wife, "I never loved you." A mother said to her daughter, "I never wanted a child." These words puncture the hearts of those who hear them. If we permit ourselves to perceive the pain we've inflicted, guilt pierces our hearts as well. Not only do we bear witness to another's suffering, but we're responsible for it. Guilt tells us that we love deeply or feel empathy for the feelings of a fellow human being. Guilt motivates us to make repairs and change our hurtful behaviors. Sometimes we cannot repair an injury due to death, distance, or other factors. The person we've wounded may not accept our apologies. But we can still change our injurious ways in future relationships. A dad might try to repair his failures with his son by showing more love to his granddaughter.

The strength to bear guilt requires self-compassion, which develops when significant others love us despite our failures. If we believe wrongdoing condemns us to damnation, how do we find the strength to face our flaws and become better people? Since guilt requires the capacity to empathize, how do we extend such understanding if we haven't received it? Tragically, many are deprived of loving attunement and must

DOI: 10.4324/9780429399633-9

overcome their shame before facing their guilt. Shame tells us we are unworthy of forgiveness and cannot change, discouraging any efforts to make amends. In despair, we may become cruel to ourselves and obsess on our shortcomings while those we've wounded recede from our awareness. Their suffering goes unattended while we are absorbed with self-hatred or defend against our guilt by denying our responsibility. Many of our clients must overcome self-loathing before they can withstand the pain of guilt and love others. Self-contempt breeds contempt for others, spawning greater wreckage. We walk away from relationships instead of tending to them and avoid the sadness or grief that comes with genuine remorse. Frequently, people suffering from chronic depression, addictions, and a host of symptoms suffer from severe unresolved guilt.

I sometimes sense guilt in my clients intuitively before I have evidence for it. Maybe someone mentions their mother, and I see the pain in their eyes. Something will prompt me to ask, "Do you feel guilty about your mother?" A phrase might telegraph guilt, such as when a man who was exploring anger toward his father said, "He's quite elderly and frail." We might wonder what does his age have to do with feeling angry at him? Very little, but the thought signals guilt for feeling angry at a man he loves who cannot defend himself. The client's anger never reaches full consciousness at great expense to himself.

Toxic vs Healthy Guilt

"Toxic guilt" is a feeling of guilt in the body, triggered by a real or imagined injury to another, fused with self-harming, defensive reactions such as self-loathing, denial, and avoidance. "As a guilt-substitute, the unconscious need for punishment should not be conflated with the guilt it evades" (Carveth, 2001). Toxic guilt blocks healthy guilt impulses to repair the relationship, involving genuine remorse with sadness or grief. Toxic guilt can arise when we condemn ourselves for aggressive impulses (which do no harm if not acted out), or we judge ourselves harshly for an inaccurate perception that we deserve blame.

We have opportunities to lessen toxic guilt and increase healthy remorse throughout every phase of the therapeutic process. We can chip away at toxic guilt in a multitude of ways, and when rage reaches consciousness, it can be less guilt-laden as a result of prior work. As healers and relievers of suffering, therapists often find it counterintuitive to encourage their clients to face the pain of healthy guilt, although growth depends upon it. One client described a horrifying act that he had committed, and I felt a thud in my heart. Neither of us wanted to face this reality. In other cases, a client had multiple affairs or verbally abused a child. Both the therapist and client may want to rationalize or minimize the damage they've inflicted. Someone once said, "The truth heals, but first it hurts like hell." Sometimes the client's guilt reminds us of our transgressions, and we want to move away. Yet, therapists need to be agents of truth.

The following exchange occurred with a troubled parent. She had previously defended against guilt about her son with intellectualization and self-loathing. Here we see an increase in her capacity to bear guilt:

Th: I wonder if instead of shutting down, we could make more space for your feelings about not being a great parent. (Her face shows a lot of pain.) And let me know what you notice in your body. I see a lot of pain.

Ct: Yeah, there is a lot of pain. I would have made different choices with the awareness I have today. I've done some things that I wouldn't do today.

Th: Yeah, I can surely say that too. I would have made a lot of different choices. (*Self-disclosing my regrets helps normalize that humans do regrettable things due to the limitations of our awareness.*)

Ct: Yeah, and it's so painful because I love him, and I wish he didn't need to suffer as much.

Th: I can feel your pain. Tell me what you regret? Can you give a couple of examples? (*Specificity is central in the process of facing feelings.*)

Ct: Umm, I think mostly about not being able to tolerate the anxiety that his suffering ignited in me. I had a lot of confusion about boundaries and never trusting my intuition. Always trying to find the perfect answer and getting frustrated if I didn't.

Th: What would you do to him?

Ct: He was a very sensitive kid and reactive to light and noises. I was a new parent and wanted to give him a lot of stimulation. I took him to "Mommy and Me" and other things. I overdid that. It wasn't what he needed. And then he's a very bright kid but also very shy. (*She spoke about a medical condition.*)

Th: So, your anxiety and driving expectations got in the way of seeing your son accurately and being responsive to him.

Ct: I was too anxious. I was very anxious.

Th: So are you saying you have guilt about causing distress for your son?

Ct: Yeah, I always had guilt about him. I was very scared. I didn't want him. I saw myself in him.

Th: It takes courage to admit that. Could we stay with your feelings there? (*She agrees.*) The pain of guilt is rising in you. Could we stay with that pain? (*She agrees.*)

Ct: Yeah. (*She cries for awhile.*)

Th: Your pain tells us you love him, and it hurts to recognize you caused him suffering. (*Her next comment reflects work we'd done in the last year.*)

Ct: Part of my guilt is also this expectation. I don't feel it as much now as I did a year ago. I felt everything was my responsibility, and if I were a perfect mom, he wouldn't have any of his problems. (*Her attempts to achieve perfection as a mother turned parenting into a burden. She rejected her son and overcompensated for her limitations by trying to control his experiences, which only added to his suffering and her guilt.*) My understanding goes beyond the intellectual now. I feel a release in my body that his happiness is not all in my power.

Th: Wonderful!

Ct: Right now, I have a bowl of goodies. I have guilt, but I have a lot of sadness next to it. Before, it was guilt and anger at myself that I wasn't good enough, and now I can just feel sad. (*Toxic guilt transforms into healthy guilt.*)

Th: Yes. Why don't we just make space for that? So you don't have to have this anxiety and self-devaluation that cuts you off from a relationship with yourself, me, and others.

Ct: It's very, it's very new actually. This feeling of being able to just be without all this extra baggage, having to make anything painful go away, to just sit with this painful feeling of sadness, of pain. I wanted him to suffer less.

Th: You want to allow the pain, just let yourself feel that? (She cries.) And I'm also wondering about what comes to you as far as a repair?

Ct: I think part of it is being aware, which I am doing now. I've told him I have regrets, but today I would be more vulnerable with him. From now on, I will show him my sadness for having hurt him. I think before, it was more from a place of putting myself down. And also needing his forgiveness, needing to hear that from him. And now I don't need that. I can just express my sadness for the pain I caused and my regret, and that's all that is important. (*This comment represents a significant shift from a focus on herself to a focus on her son, which reparation requires.*)

Th: You're not going to be looking to him to take away your pain.

Ct: Right, right.

Th: Just like you were expecting yourself to take away his pain (*Ct: Yeah*). You're not going to expect him to take away yours (*Ct: Right*). You and I know the pain comes from a deep love for him. Your parents never allowed you to have limitations, and maybe you did not want your son because you knew you wouldn't do it perfectly. I wonder if we can also have compassion for you, as you do for your son?

Ct: Yes. I think I must.

Th: How is that feeling? To be able to talk to him and not need anything from him?

Ct: It feels like I'm creating a lot more freedom for myself and making everything so much easier. Making things easier for me to experience. It just widens my world of experiencing. I feel clear.

Therapists ask, "How are you able to make tough interventions that trigger pain, even agony?" I do it because I must, knowing that avoidance brings more suffering. If I tell myself guilt is "too much" for the client to bear and avoid doing my best work, I feel guilt too. However, I must have compassion for myself to become a better therapist. I seek a place within me that accepts my failures or inadequacies so I can find the strength to allow my clients to face theirs.

Self-Punishment

Of course, no one sets out to punish himself. The terms "self-attack" and "self-punishment" infer choice and agency to many who hear this language, which can sound accusatory to our clients. Therefore, I would use the terms "self-attack" and "self-punishment" carefully, being sure the client understands that we are not referring to something done consciously or intentionally. My exchange with Jon Frederickson sheds light on the topic of self-punishment:

> Since all defenses are initially unconscious, agency is not a factor. The child's adaptations are a way to sustain an attachment with a parent who may be chaotic, unreliable, or threatening. Self-punishment is an effect of an adaptive survival mechanism, an archaic practice that hurts oneself to avoid more unbearable suffering. It's the lesser of two evils. The child cannot contain overwhelming emotional waves and excruciating aloneness. And so, the child develops defenses to stop or distract from the pain. In trauma, the person the child turns to for help is the one inflicting pain. Unable to depend on a parent, the child must rely on defense. So he turns the rage toward the parent onto himself to re-establish the insecure attachment he needs for his survival. Thus, the defense's purpose is to regulate the parent and preserve the attachment (Sullivan; Bowlby). The defenses do not have the purpose of self-punishment, even though that is their effect. The child's defenses ward off the rage and pain the parent cannot bear, and they ward off the unbearable pain of aloneness in the insecure attachment where he must rely on defense instead of a person.
>
> (Jon Frederickson, personal communication, August 23, 2020)

When we consider that "The defenses do not have the purpose of self-punishment even though that is their effect," we see how little the person has to do with their habits of self-punishment. There is no developed "self" to inflict "self" punishment. Self-punishment is compulsive, automatic, unconscious and learned from the modeling of caregivers. Breaking habits of self-punishment requires the conscious awareness of old patterns and recognition of their alternatives, a new love for ourselves, and the experience of an attachment relationship that thrives without the need for self-punishment.

Guilt for Harm to Oneself

I may ask a client, "How do you feel about these learned habits of neglecting yourself all these years?" Clients often bring up this sad reality without prompting. We have a responsibility to ourselves just as we have to other people. Guilt for how we've treated ourselves helps people to become kinder to themselves. Some clients say that it's next to impossible to step outside themselves and see themselves as separate people, but we need this perspective to develop a relationship to ourselves. Who hasn't been nasty toward themselves in ways we'd never direct to another person? Why do we feel free to talk to ourselves like we're subhuman? Often, we're barely aware of this activity. It's very hopeful when people connect to their guilt for ignoring, loathing, and depriving themselves. Imagine patting one hand on top of your other hand and saying soothingly to yourself, "Hey, it's good you feel guilt for allowing your suffering. You're worthy of better care. You deserve your tears. How would you want to treat yourself differently in the future?"

Guilt is an Emotion—Development and Physiology of Guilt

Guilt activates feelings in the body. When we commit an act and see the pain in the eyes of the other and grasp the link between the two, guilt arises. Guilt is a stressful event. The ability to recognize this feeling and repair injuries to others may be the single most valuable relationship skill we can possess. We have to be able to heal ruptures to have secure relationships in our lives. Some researchers have identified guilt at 36 months (Izard, 1978; Schore, 1994; Sroufe, 1979), and others report guilt at eight years (Ferguson et al., 1991). In the following study, researchers believed guilt to be recognizable as an emotion at 22 months:

> ... when they believed they had committed a transgression, children as young as 22 months showed a highly coherent response that reflected tension. That tension was expressed by gaze aversion, multiple bodily signals, increased negative and suppressed positive emotion, and overall appearance of being affected by the event. (Kochanska et al., 2002)

When we help our clients become familiar with the areas of the body that signal specific emotions, we help them to identify what they are feeling. Damasio said, "Emotions are not subjective, not private, not elusive, not intangible, not indefinable. Their neurobiology can be investigated objectively, and understanding their neurobiology opens the way to elucidating the neurobiology of feelings" (Damasio, 2004, p. 56). Since others may see and perceive our emotions, we are at a distinct disadvantage when we cannot recognize them, causing our communications to lack congruity. "Why is she smiling when she sounds angry?" "Why did he say he had a great time, but he looks so sad?" Knowledge of the physiology of emotions helps the therapist to attune to the client's emotional experiences and guide them to identify what they feel accurately. Toxic and healthy guilt share two common factors: the neurobiology of guilt and the belief we have injured another, though we may deny it. When the feeling of guilt is driven from consciousness, it continues to exist within our bodies alongside the defenses against it. Just as the feeling of anger is different from the defense of verbal discharge or acting out, both involve the same neurobiology (e.g., activation in the solar plexus) with similar triggers (e.g., a reaction to a psychological injury) (see Figure 2.1).

I found it difficult to access information and agreement on guilt's physiology and sought clarification from Allan Abbass, MD, Professor, and Director at Dalhousie University in Halifax, Canada, and Doug Kahn, MD, Clinical Professor of Psychiatry, University of California, Irvine. Dr. Abbass and Dr. Kahn frequently work with guilt over rage. Dr. Abbass has observed an intensely painful feeling with tears associated with injuring an attachment figure, involving constriction of the upper chest, larynx, pharynx, and neck muscles (personal communication, October, 05, 2020). Dr. Kahn found that his patients, "to a person, described guilt as a fleeting but distinct sensation of nausea (some mentioning 'disgust' and a 'sick feeling') always felt in the epigastrium, but clearly distinct, in their experience, from any nausea they have ever felt from anxiety or other causes" (personal communication, December, 7, 2020). I tracked guilt in my body after I had wounded a friend inadvertently. I had a distinct sickening feeling around the diaphragm and upper abdomen, which is the epigastrium area. Our bodies can give us great information on the neurobiology of emotions.

To Deactivate Toxic Guilt, Activate the Healing Triad

Awareness of Guilt

This client denies that his aggressive behavior hurts others and thereby avoids the self-condemnation that he has linked to guilt. He must become aware of this dynamic before he can change it.

Th: Jack, you say that your mother overreacted when you yelled at her. She may have overreacted, but wouldn't we assume she was also hurt? How do you feel about yelling at her?

Ct: I don't think it was a big deal. (*Avoidance, minimization, rationalization.*)

Th: I realize you see it that way. I wonder what happens inside you if you registered that you hurt your mother?

Ct: That wouldn't be ok. Only a bad person would do that.

Th: Does this mean that if you were to do something you'd want to correct, then your entire person becomes unacceptable? Do you condemn all of you for some parts of you?

Ct: I never looked at this.

Th: How does it feel to look at this?

Ct: It gives me some relief. It never occurred to me that I could act like a jerk and still be a decent person.

Th: I'm glad you're seeing that you're neither all good or bad but rather a flawed human who has value. As an alternative to assuming you'd be a "bad person," we could look at your feelings toward your mother right before you yelled at her, so you don't have to dismiss your feelings or hers. Your anger at her feels unacceptable to you, so you discharge your anger rapidly. I wonder if we could look at the fact that you were angry, lashed out, and hurt her without condemning yourself? Then, we could help you.

Jack operates under a system that has no tolerance for his flaws and failures. Self-loathing underlies his denial of guilt. He reflexively blames others who protest his behaviors because he can't bear his flaws.

The Therapeutic Transfer of Compassion for Self

Jack will continue to act out (yelling) until he recognizes his defense of splitting. If he owns that he hurt his mother, he becomes "all bad" in his mind. He will have to accept his flaws, which requires self-compassion, before taking responsibility and facing his guilt. I attempt to awaken compassion for the suffering caused by his internal harsh critic.

Th: You had intense feelings toward your mother and your feelings deserve to be recognized. But when you act out by blowing up, it harms both of you. It seems like an internal bully makes no space for you to feel your anger. You must get rid of your anger immediately. And this bully would condemn you if you were to consider that you hurt your mother. How tragic!

Ct: You're saying that I'm not a bad person if I hurt my mother?

Th: Your actions don't define you, and you can make repairs. But you will continue to hurt others and yourself if we don't make some room to acknowledge your rage.

We hope to generate compassion for the cost of repressing his complex feelings. Toxic guilt often involves splitting. If we are either a person who loves or a person who wants to destroy and we can't be both, we will feel guilty for our feelings. Do we not all struggle with this dichotomy? Paradoxically, if this man accepted his impulses to lash out, he wouldn't be lashing out.

The Will

The self-condemnation that fuels toxic guilt transforms through the desire to release the chains that bind our feelings. Without the will to care, therapy stands still. This man loved his mother and also acted out his rage. If he continues to deny this reality, he will never have the tools to repair his relationships or work through his feelings. Our clients desperately need to recognize the specific damage caused to them and others due to self-condemnation (a prison term with no release date). And they need to care about that damage. I could never help a man who had had 26 courses of electroshock therapy for chronic depression. He couldn't or wouldn't release his guilt for his mother's suicide because he had wished her dead.

We will see the power of will with Dennis, a passionate and gifted screenwriter. He almost died from cocaine, but thankfully he is in recovery. When he spoke of his mother, she was always the good and perfect parent. Whenever we approached his feelings toward her, he'd draw a blank. Paradoxically, he repressed his rage at her, yet he stabbed her in the heart by never visiting her. Since his mother had been his life-support growing up, Dennis found it impossible to allow angry feelings toward her. In therapy, he found more strength to stop running from his emotions. The following session, a turning point in his treatment, helped free him from his defense of repression so he could face his fury at his mother and his unconscious toxic guilt for his impulses to destroy her. As he became more integrated, he started visiting his aging mother (Warshow 2002).

Ct: Guess I'm at a point where it's easier for me to look back and hold her responsible for the lack of guidance and consideration for me, especially with the number of times we moved. I just got my high school transcripts the other day. They were terrible. D's and F's. (*Yet he is an intelligent, capable man.*)

Th: You were floundering on your own.

Ct: Yeah. And I thought, "I can't show these to anybody." I'm embarrassed. There was a point when we moved from Denver to Boise, and I didn't have any money, but I made a punching bag. I realize now I was furious. (*It's a great sign when a client recovers memories and recognizes trauma-related feelings for the first time.*)

Th: I'm so glad you're remembering.

Ct: And I'd go down to the basement and punch on it all the time. I would also get into fights.

Th: Who were you punching?

Ct: That's just it. At the time, I didn't know who I was punching.

Th: Hm, Hmm. What about now?

Ct: Well, yeah. I was definitely punching my mom. You know, I look at the crappy decisions that she made and how she ignored me. So many frickin' times we moved. (*She also was passive when his father became violent.*) It was easier for her to leave and try somewhere else than to stay and slug it out.

For the first time, he stopped rationalizing his mother's behavior and allowed himself to feel violent impulses coursing through his body, accompanied by a brutal fantasy. These impulses had lived inside him since early childhood. Ultimately he hurled his mother over a cliff in a fantasy, which brought him tremendous relief. Then the process slowed due to guilt over his rage. Avoiding guilt had poisoned him for years. We needed to face it together.

Th: How wonderful you could be free to have your true feelings at last. I'm also aware that your emotions toward your mom are complex. You've described her tenderness and how her voice could melt you. When you let yourself feel that love between you, what do you feel about your violent impulses toward her?

Guilt over rage frequently shows up at this juncture because the client also loves his mother. Therapists who enter this terrain with their clients need to be prepared to explore for guilt. The client must integrate his loving feelings, which he'd previously denied by acting out and not visiting her. When guilt over mixed feelings of love and rage is overlooked, the guilt may incite more self-punishment and defenses. We don't want a client to leave a session with unaddressed guilt over rage. It can lead to a bad outcome. Dennis responds to my probing inquiry into his complex emotions:

Ct: I'm sorry. I just feel sorry. I'm sorry, Mom (*grunts, rocking*). I'm sorry I hurt you. (*His remorse expresses his love. The guilt rises because he can now feel love toward the mother he wanted to kill. The more he can feel this guilt, the less he will have to punish himself for this "crime."*)

Th: You care deeply. There's remorse. As you feel love for her are you aware of any other impulses?

Ct: Hold her. Hold and rock her (*makes more rocking movements*).

Th: What's her response to you as you're rocking her and holding her?

Ct: She'd pat me (*said with a whisper.*) She'd pat me and say, "That's okay, honey. It's okay." (*Starts to sob deeply.*)

Th: She'd have compassion for you. She would forgive you.

Ct: (*Deep, wailing sobs, rocking back and forth*).

Th: Tell me about your grief. (*After a prolonged period of sobbing passes.*)

Ct: (*Whispers*) Just to say that I was sorry. Would you forgive me? She says there's nothing to forgive.

Th: She understands, and she even realizes how you could have such rage toward her. She accepts you for who you are. Do you, Dennis?

Ct: I always wanted to make up excuses for her.

Th: And deny your rageful impulses toward her and your reality. And how do you feel now about that aggressive part?

Ct: I like that part. I like feeling strong. I like feeling powerful. I know I'm a good person. I've been ignoring the good part. I'm looking at it out of balance and using that as an excuse to punish myself. Because the program says that when you're guilty, you have to punish yourself. If you're bad, punishment follows.

His statement validates his right to feel rage, which protested the extreme deprivation of his needs. In the following exploration, the client discovered that he had childhood fears that he would lose control of his rage like his father, end up in jail, and be unloved. These unconscious anxieties were no longer a concern. He saw that he'd anesthetized himself with cocaine to numb the pain, acute anxiety, excruciating sense of unworthiness, and aloneness. He'd treated himself with the indifference, neglect, and cruelty that he learned from his parents. His unconscious murderous feelings turned into self-hatred and self-punishment.

He felt relieved that he could have violent impulses and complex feelings toward his mother without destroying his loving feelings for her or seeing himself as a bad person. The holidays followed soon after this session. Dennis had not planned to be with his mother. Instead he drove out of state to visit his mother and even painted her home for days. He was pleased with his accomplishment. He and his brother lounged on the couch together, and his brother slid his head onto Dennis's shoulder. I almost gasped. His older brother had tortured him as a kid, and Dennis hated him. They talked together about their childhood truthfully for the first time. A warm feeling filled my chest. They'd found each other again! During the termination session, I asked Dennis how he felt about his course of therapy? He replied, "I'm giving myself an A." His comment delighted us both, considering he once talked disparagingly about his D's and F's in school. He'd made the grade!

Guilt is a Moral Emotion

Guilt has been described as a "moral emotion" (Tangney et al., 2007) and would not exist without the ability to intuit and care about another's experience. Guilt requires mentalization, enabling us to grasp another's psychological state and empathize with others' feelings. We know there is severe psychological damage when guilt is absent or greatly diminished in the personality. Therefore, we want to encourage awareness of harm to others and also increase mentalization, the awareness of the internal experience of another. For example:

Th: So that's what happened when you were working in the office with your husband? You felt angry at him that he wasn't moving faster?

Ct: Understanding faster, yeah.

Th: He wasn't doing things the way you wanted him to?

Ct: Yeah.

Th: Which seems like a common theme between you, attacking him for his shortcomings, doesn't it? (*She agrees.*) And you link that to your mother. That's how she treated you?

Ct: Yeah, yes.

Th: And how do you feel when you see yourself falling into that same pattern?

Ct: I'm having a hard time connecting. I think I must be having a lot of grief and sadness around it. (*She blames and judges others reflexively as her mother devalued her. She has difficulty staying with the pain of her guilt for hurting her husband.*)

Th: Tell me about the grief that you're aware of (*focusing on avoided guilt*).

Ct: The grief I'm aware of happened as I was in this mode, and I saw what it was doing to him, but I needed to punish him too, you know? And I think it's really sad that I do that to him when he's very innocent in all of this.

Th: So the anger that comes up in you when he's not responding satisfactorily turns to abuse? (*Calling it what it is*).

Ct: Yes, it feels abusive. And it feels like it looks for reasons to be that way. It's like it's hunting for a whipping post.

Th: It's good you can acknowledge that. How does it feel to say that?

Ct: It feels good to keep recognizing that, and it feels good to acknowledge that with you. Because I don't want to sit in the dark with it by myself.

We work to name the avoided feelings

Th: Let's see if we can identify your feelings. Are you aware of feeling guilty about this?

Ct: You know, I don't connect to a lot of guilt and remorse, and I think that's where I need help. My experience is that when I can connect to my sadness or really see what's happening to the other person, then I feel more connected to myself. I feel more connected to myself when I can feel the sadness.

Th: I would think so. I want to encourage you to let yourself feel your sadness.

Ct: Yeah. First, I connect to my own helplessness. (*She was helpless to get her needs met by her mother. She learned to act out her anger like her mother, and she feels powerless in the face of the habit.*) It's like, "Oh, that's what she trained me to do. And that is what I do when I'm triggered, or something snaps in me." It feels good to acknowledge that happens for me. (*Connecting to the observing part of herself is powerfully liberating. We are not our habits.*)

Th: It's excellent for you to talk to me about this pattern. And you're also speaking to this innocence in him—that he is just being who he is—a human with limitations.

Ct: Right.

Confronting the reality of inflicting harm on another

Th: And now you recognize that your devaluations inflict pain and suffering for him?

Ct: Yes.

Th: And then you notice there is a part of you that lusts after and finds pleasure in his suffering.

Ct: Yes.

I did not invite her to go deeper into her sadness and the pain of her guilt because she had been re-enacting an early trauma. We had to explore her compulsive, sadistic impulses before she could connect to feelings of guilt. We needed to clear a space for her rage at her mother to pass through first.

Th: How about if we keep exploring that part that finds pleasure and see what it has to express?

Ct: Yeah, it's very much like a predator, and that's how it's getting satisfaction, and that's its way of asserting power or control. I think it's even more primal than that. It's just dark and sadistic.

Th: What if you allow it to come out here, and we could invite this sadistic part and see how it would feel like inflicting pain on him if it could fully express itself?

Ct: OK.

After her rage filled her body and she released its impulses, she became aware she'd been re-enacting trauma with her mother. In her rage fantasy, she expressed her drive to reclaim her power by sadistically dominating him, as her mother sadistically dominated her. She sees that her rage has nothing to do with him. As the session comes to a close, she expresses her remorse and deep pain for hurting her spouse. She intends to apologize to him, and she expresses her will to overcome her sadism.

"Consolidate the Dichotomy" of Complex Feelings

Unconscious self-punishment could take the form of a substance disorder, social anxiety, or depression, all of which plagued Paul, a talented man in his thirties. Toxic guilt prevented him from facing his hatred toward his parents, and I'd never worked with anyone with stronger defenses against his rage. When he showed a flash of anger and I noticed it, he lashed out at me for making something up. Denial of feelings can gaslight others, causing others to doubt their reality. Working with him challenged my ability to trust my perceptions and stand by them. After considerable work with the denial of his anger, he surprised me. He pulled out the screensaver on his phone with a sad photo of him at 7 years old, a daily reminder of his trauma and unresolved guilt.

He points to the picture of himself:

Ct: That is my birthday. I'm not happy. I'm smiling for the camera because my mom told me to do this.

Th: May I see it? (*He passes the phone to me. I see the face of a child in despair. I groan.*)

Ct: I'd asked to have three friends over to celebrate my birthday. The excuse my mom gave me was there's no room in the house. I came to realize that she was embarrassed by our place so no one could visit me.

His mother's shame and self-absorption caused her to ignore her son's feelings and needs habitually. Even more egregious, she did not protect him from his violent father and step-father. The birthday incident was one disappointment among countless others.

Th: That's terrible, Paul! What a loss for the little boy that you were. Do you want to say what you're feeling?

Ct: Just a lot of sadness for what could have been.

Th: Oh, I feel so sad too.

Ct: I still haven't forgiven her, and I'm sad for myself that I'm not able to let that go. There's a lot of shame for feeling that kind of resentment and anger. Like I, I'm ashamed that I don't want to pick up the phone and call my mom or spend time with her. I'm ashamed that I want to distance myself from my family.

He feels a lot of guilt because he knows his withdrawal tortures his mother and deprives his siblings. He is unconsciously anxious he'll lose control of his feelings when he is in his mother's presence. He redirects his rage toward himself in the form of shame. As I've said, trauma feelings are like children standing at the door, waiting for someone to let them in. They do not go quietly into the night.

Th: I hear that you care about your family very much, but why should we direct shame toward this innocent boy? (*My voice filled with compassion.*) Why should he be condemned for his hurt and inevitable anger? (*Anger is the flip side of hurt.*)

Ct: It makes me a bad son for being angry at his mom.

Th: He's bad for having feelings when he doesn't get to have his friends over, and he's alone on his birthday? Does he have to hide who he is? And where he lives? He's supposed to be a "good boy?"

Ct: But it's my mommy (*he begins to cry*).

Th: Why shouldn't this boy have the right to all his feelings? I know he loves his mommy. But why can't he have all his feelings?

Ct: Because that makes him a bad boy. She doesn't deserve to be on the receiving end of that. (*He begins to sob. His guilt for his rage is toxic, but his guilt for neglecting his mother is healthy.*)

Th: Yeah, a bad boy. Mm. Just let it come. It's okay. Very painful. If you and I create a place where you can have your feelings here, how do you harm your mother? Tell me about your tears. (*He then describes healthy remorse for acting out his retaliatory rage and causing her to suffer.*)

Ct: The tears came from the fact that I can't stand to be around my family. The pain that I know she's in, from how I've been managing my anger toward her. And that's from a distance. (*He had integrated the fact that he deals with his anger destructively by avoidance and withdrawal.*) My pain comes from being unable to show my Mom how much I love her because of how furious I am.

Th: What if I told you that I think we could get to the place you want if you make space for your feelings? I see no way around them.

Ct: No. I was just remembering. When my uncle died, I saw my family for the first time in two years. And I hated every second of it.

Th: You know, that child is not going to go quietly into the night (*pointing to the little boy pictured on his iPhone who never got to have his feelings*).

Ct: Sometimes, I wish he would (*a tragic rejection of the child he was*).

Th: How is it feeling sharing this enormous pain with me?

Ct: A little cathartic. The adult in me is extremely grateful and empathetic toward my Mom, all she sacrificed for me. The adult in me feels guilty. The child hates my mom for what she put me through and how she raised me, and what a messed-up individual I am because of her.

Th: You have lots of different feelings that are natural and unavoidable. Do your feelings have to cancel each other out? (*I'm encouraging Paul to bear his rage and complex feelings, so he does not have to split them apart and deny his humanity and his love.*)

Ct: I guess I want to learn how to—consolidate the dichotomy of it.

Th: Oh! I'm so on board with helping you to do that! You've had enough of being a false self. Your mom felt it was necessary, but it's the last thing you want. And if we're going to be our true selves, you and I both have a whole range of feelings toward people we love. (*Normalizing complex feelings*). And it doesn't mean we're not grateful. It doesn't mean we don't love deeply. All of our emotions have a right to exist.

Ct: I just want to consolidate the dichotomy.

In the session following this one, the client acknowledged the full intensity of his annihilatory rage toward his mother, that felt like "destroying cities" and "blowing up buildings." He'd been terrified of losing control of his rage, so he was very relieved to discover his capacity to feel rage without harming anyone. In the months that followed, he landed and sustained the best job of his life and was able to work through conflicts in the workplace directly and productively for the first time. He consciously works to maintain a state of self-compassion and has said his suicidal ideation is non-existent. He is no longer in a vegetative depression. This final vignette from a pre-termination session after he had visited his family showed us his efforts to repair the splitting:

Ct: Like, I had a good time (*with his family*).

Th: Wow!

Ct: Because that was one of the first real conversations we'd ever had. I was like, "Look, let's put this family dynamic BS aside for a second and act like we're just all adults." And that turned out to be a really good experiment. We started having fun and laughing and enjoying each other.

Th: I celebrate for you because I know you've carried guilt about avoiding your mother.

Ct: Yeah. And I don't have that fear that caused me to avoid her anymore. I don't have the shame for not wanting to talk to her. I'm reacting to a lot of stuff differently. I'm not immediately sliding into the "less than" category in the back of my head.

Let's take a look at the trajectory that landed Paul in a place of profound healing. The Healing Triad guided my responses. We began with raising awareness of the obstacles to his feelings, activating compassion for his suffering due to those protective barriers, and mobilizing his will to risk self-exposure. The unconscious alliance prompted him to reveal a photo of himself as a child, with his traumas etched on his face. He wanted to banish this child for his fury toward his mother, but he allowed my compassion to penetrate and overpower his contempt for himself. He faced the truth that he both loved and hated his mother, which gave way to an amazing desire to "consolidate the dichotomy" of his conflicted feelings. His will allowed his volcanic rage to break through to consciousness, so that he could resolve his guilt and shame. I don't believe we would have arrived at this quality of connection without shame sensitivity, building safety that I would not humiliate him.

Signs that Toxic Guilt Needs Attention

We can diminish toxic guilt one exchange at a time, like water chipping away at a stone. Overlooking guilt in therapy is common, so we need to sharpen our antennas. Numerous clients who have worked with toxic guilt in therapy said that the guilt dissolved within a session, never to return. I primarily draw my conclusions about the efficacy of the work from my client's feedback, healthy changes in their lives, and other people's validation of their progress. I have observed that my clients resolve toxic guilt in a variety of ways, including those mentioned in the list below. May we open our minds to the complexity of healing, so we do not accept a one-size-fits-all remedy. Many different kinds of interventions can make a real difference in helping our clients heal from toxic guilt. Sometimes embodied compassion can be more powerful than words in facilitating the release of toxic guilt. I suggest we keep an eye on the following indicators of toxic guilt:

1 Feelings suddenly shut down despite a strong alliance
2 Feelings, impulses, and fantasies are confused with deeds
3 Denial or minimization of causing harm to others
4 Tolerance for cruelty toward oneself
5 A belief that feeling anger is wrong
6 Surviving when others weren't so lucky
7 Undeserved guilt
8 Absorbing another's negative projections
9 Denial of the pain caused by unconscious defenses
10 Repressive defenses against healthy guilt

Feelings Shut Down Despite a Strong Alliance

A client risks telling me about her cruelty toward her little sister when they were children. She suddenly detaches:

Th: As you were taking the risk of describing your cruelty to your little sister, darkness settled over you. I wonder if you felt guilty and went numb so as not to feel the pain of what you did to her?

Ct: I can't believe how I bullied her (*head in hands, commingling of shame and guilt*). She didn't deserve it.

Th: I'm sure you're right. Emotionally abusing your younger sister is extremely tough to admit. (*This response confirms the harsh reality and may be difficult for the therapist to state. I want to resist the temptation to minimize.*) You're expressing your caring right now. I suggest you allow yourself to stay with this painful feeling.

Ct: How could I do that to her?

Th: We can get to that. I'm sure there was a reason. How about if we stay with your pain for now, as you experience your love for your little sister. Your pain tells us how much you care.

Feelings, Impulses, and Fantasies are Confused with Deeds

"Due to the immaturity of the child's mind, she often feels her wish is the same as a deed. Operating in concrete-operational thought (Piaget), she equates a wish with a deed. So she keeps feeling guilty for wishes she never acted out" (Frederickson, 2012).

Sexual fantasies and Guilt

An endearing young man tortured himself with self-doubt and blame because of momentary sexual arousal while holding his son. I explored in-depth if any acting out had occurred or if he feared losing control of his impulses. He said his sexual feeling had been brief, and he never touched his son inappropriately. He was sure he never would. I believed him. I spoke with Alexandra Katehakis, the Clinical Director of the Center for Healthy Sex, and she commented on his concerns:

> The difference between those who offend —whether covertly or overtly—and those who don't is that those who don't talk about their fantasies to someone (partner, therapist, friend, etc.). It's perfectly normal for parents to have these feelings. Children are sexual, beautiful, guileless, and evoke arousal in us. Novelty and arousal are just that. It's the meaning we give to the arousal and the firing of sexual

> fantasy that creates guilt. Shame and guilt in these cases are prosocial functions; morality, values, and conscience are on board for those who don't offend.
>
> (Personal communication, November 15, 2020)

In another instance, a woman says she feels guilty because of a sexual fantasy about a coworker. If she obsesses about her fantasies and distances herself from her husband to torture herself for her imagination, she harms her marriage. A momentary fantasy does not warrant guilt and guilt never warrants self-punishment.

Guilt over rage impulses

- Normalize rage by pointing out its survival and hard-wired retaliatory aspects.
  "It's natural to feel like retaliating when you're wounded."
  "When we're injured, we're hard-wired to respond in equal measure."
- Point out that no one is harmed by a rage impulse in the body. Challenge irrational ideas about rage. Explain the difference between acting out and feeling an emotion.
  "It's just us in the room. We cannot damage anyone by a thought or internal experience of a feeling."
- Explain the real damage when toxic guilt blocks rage, causing rage to be acted out or internalized.
- Highlight that guilt arises over rage only when we care about the other person. Hence, guilt is a sign of our capacity to love.
- Raise awareness that the client can feel rage and be a loving person. Rage and love do not cancel each other out.
- Convey that the client and therapist together can manage rage in the service of healing.

Researchers have found that guilt-laden grief following an intense breakthrough to rage is a path to a positive outcome (Abbass & Town, 2013; Abbass et al., 2017). Allowing rage and love to release from the body causes anxiety to drop and allows for the integration of internal conflicts. The impending pain of guilt has been considered the motive force for conscious resistance to breakthroughs in intensive dynamic therapy (Davanloo, 2000). Accessing guilt over rage is one powerful path to healing toxic guilt, as I've illustrated in vignettes.

People ask, "Why doesn't this person have more intense guilt following a breakthrough to rage?" Skill development is one factor. Also, the grip of toxic guilt over feelings may have lessened in numerous prior interactions with the therapist. After a rage breakthrough, a man said, "I deserve to have my feelings. I do not feel guilty about them. I feel a lot of compassion for that kid who had to endure so much abuse. His feelings did not harm anyone. I no longer feel guilty for my anger." He sobbed for the pain he'd endured as a child. A client may recognize that they don't have intensely conflicted feelings, including love toward a mom or dad who was viciously abusive. Conflicted feelings are typically more intense toward figures that expressed love. I recall a story in which Davanloo pointed out the significance of a tear that rolled down a man's cheek after a breakthrough to rage.

Denial and Minimization of Causing Harm to Others

One of my clients told me she'd had a lengthy affair, and when her husband found out, he hung himself. She recounted the story with little feeling, and she had been chronically depressed since he died. Internally, I was horrified and readily understood why she numbed her guilt and disappeared into a void of empty words. When she denied her guilt, I replied:

> *Th:* Everything you say in our session has significance, and I'm aware you are telling me about this tragic event because you have feelings about it. Yet your words seem disconnected from your feelings. It must be hard to tell me that your actions contributed to your husband's suicide. The cost of pushing your feelings aside kills off something in you too. (*Her eyes filled with tears, and a path opened to explore both her rage and grief over the fact that she rarely felt loved by her husband, nor had she shown love toward him.*)

Jon Frederickson presented a session with a man who had shattered numerous women's lives through his negligence, dishonesty, and cruel devaluation. Without access to guilt, he could not sustain a relationship.

In therapy, the client revealed that he had tortured a cat as a child. Jon unflinchingly guided him to relive the suffering he had inflicted on this poor creature. The man began to rock with sobs for a prolonged period. The session was tough to watch. Jon helped this man face guilt for his callousness toward the cat and the women in his life. The man began making repairs in his current relationships. Redemption required him to take this journey of thorns. I was deeply moved by this man's passage from inhumane to human, as he discovered his capacity to care.

The AA 12 Steps says it well: "Made direct amends to such people wherever possible, except when to do so would injure them or others." And "The readiness to take the full consequences of our past acts, and to take responsibility for the well-being of others at the same time, is the very spirit of Step Nine" (*Twelve steps and twelve traditions*, 1989, p. 83). I was profoundly touched when a former client, who had joined an AA program, made an appointment to see me because she wanted to make amends for something she'd said to me. The capacity to bear the pain of full remorse and make amends often begins with intensive work to transcend shame and self-loathing. We need a sense of worth to acknowledge our flaws. Otherwise, we'll engage in splitting and denial of our guilt because we must be all good or else we'll collapse into self-condemnation because we're all bad. We won't have the inner space to recognize our mix of strengths and weaknesses. We have to have a sense of self before we can take responsibility without self-condemnation. Staying compassionately connected to our flawed humanity gives us the inner strength to reach out to the injured other, sincerely and wholeheartedly apologize, and repair the injury. Healing from guilt also requires our efforts to make long-term changes in the behaviors that wounded others. Those clients brave enough to acknowledge their wrongdoings to others in a deeply caring way move me deeply. I tell them so.

Tolerance for Cruelty toward Oneself

As a daughter explores rage at her abusive mom, she feels guilt:

Ct: But my mom's father used to beat her too, and her family was very poor. She had it worse than me. She doesn't deserve my anger.

Th: I appreciate that you have a lot of empathy for mom, despite her lashing you with a belt numerous times. But where is the compassion for that young child who has feelings about the agony she endured? I feel pain for her, believing that she was worthless, rather than understanding it was her mom who acted shamelessly. Perhaps your guilt for your feelings toward your mom inflicts the ultimate cruelty on yourself. (*Silence*). How is it to hear my words?

Ct: It's terrible when I think about it. I've been discounting myself for many years and feel really sad for all I've lost. I have to stop treating myself this way.

When people begin to heal, they often break through the denial of the pain and loss caused by defensive patterns. There is value in feeling healthy remorse for cruelties toward ourselves. Our clients may need to grieve the suffering they would have been spared if they had possessed their new awareness years ago. Why should we show any less compassion for depriving ourselves than we would for hurting a loved one? Just as we have the opportunity to repair relationships with others, we can repair our relationship with ourselves.

A Belief that Feeling Anger is Wrong

Identification with an out-of-control parent, leading to guilt over rage:

Ct: Anger is destructive.

Th: Your parents lost control and acted out their anger, and that was horribly destructive to you and your siblings. However, in its pure form, anger is energy in your body that does not harm anyone. Does it seem fair to carry guilt for a feeling you never acted out? Your parent's anger didn't hurt you. The ways they acted out their anger hurt you. You've tried to repress your anger all your life. Where has that taken you? I see only depression. Instead, might we allow you to experience your feelings freely?

Dealing with guilt over anger:

Ct: I know my boyfriend left me a few times, but isn't it wrong to have anger toward someone who is so damaged?

Th: How about the damage that is done to you when your anger is abandoned? (*My language and tone intend to evoke sympathy.*)

Ct: Are you saying I might make different choices with men if I had more access to my anger? (*She'd been involved with an addict and a man who had serial affairs.*)

Th: Think of a cat without claws in a neighborhood where predators roam. (*Love those metaphors!*)

Misdirected guilt:

Ct: (*Looking away from me*). Umm, I ran away from home when I was 14 because my mother abused me for the first 14 years of my life, physically abused me.

Th: Oh, how tragic! How traumatic.

Ct: I mean, literally, I was in fear for my life, day and night. She would throw me against the corner of the wall. (*Th: Oh!*) She pulled my hair, hit me, and told me that she would kill me if I cried. (*She begins to hyperventilate.*)

Th: Barbara, can you just look at me, can you just be aware that I'm here with you? And that you're not at the mercy of your mother anymore? (*She looks at me for an extended period and becomes less terrified. After her anxiety subsided, she resumed.*)

Ct: I hated her. Hated her. And even today, God says you have to forgive. It's tough. I say I've forgiven her, but I don't know that I have. I just hope that God hasn't let her get off the hook. (*Mother is deceased.*)

Th: I believe the anger you have is there for a reason, and when you try to push it away, or you judge yourself, you can hardly breathe, you get foggy and overwhelmed. Is that what you want for yourself?

Ct: No, I don't. So you think it's okay if I just say that she was an awful person and that I hated her for what she did to me?

Th: It's not only ok; it's vital. (*She went on to have a massive breakthrough of rage and later was able to have a surprisingly tender relationship with her mother.*) (Warshow, 2003).

Surviving When Others Weren't So Lucky

A sister felt guilty because she got straight A's while her little brother was barely passing. She felt ashamed and restricted around him:

Ct: When I see him, I remember how much he suffered because my parents got excited when I got my grades. Especially when I got into a top university. How can I feel good about my accomplishments when he couldn't do what I could do?

Th: Hey, I know, it's a shame your brother had to struggle so much in school. I'm feeling for you, too, because you couldn't celebrate your accomplishments joyously, and that was a significant loss! Wouldn't his struggles have existed whether you were born or not? He has immense value regardless of his limitations, and I hope your parents helped him feel that. Your guilt causes you to hide your feelings from him to this day. What if your guilt, rather than your gifts, is the most significant cause of suffering in your relationship with your brother today?

Undeserved Guilt

Causing discomfort to others does not always warrant guilt. Pain can serve growth or stunt it. We need to make a distinction. A client felt guilt for creating discomfort when she told a friend she felt hurt that her friend barely acknowledges her at social events. She's would like to be treated differently and is not blaming or accusing her friend. She is making a good faith effort to strengthen their friendship. It would be great if her friend makes amends and tries a little harder. The shame and guilt her friend might experience may help her grow.

Excessive guilt:

Ct: My mother wouldn't have fallen and injured herself if I hadn't left my bike outside. I can never forgive myself. I've been so upset and distracted that I'm not paying attention to my daughter.

Th: I can imagine how terrible you must feel! I'd feel horrible, too, because you love your mom. But if your 8-year-old daughter left her bike outside, would she deserve such extreme condemnation?

Ct: No, of course not.

Th: But you deserve harsher treatment for an oversight? Might your guilt be excessively cruel to you and causing more suffering for your family?

Ct: I see that I treat myself differently, and I don't know why.

Th: Do you see that condemning yourself for your mom's accident is highly damaging? Would you want to allow yourself to feel sadness for your mother's injury without needing to blame yourself, so you don't also have to feel guilty for neglecting your daughter?

Ct: How do I do that?

Th: You would need to feel compassion for your suffering, as I do. (*I am silent to create space for her to feel my compassion.*) Is it your will to show caring for yourself and release this guilt that doesn't belong to you?

Ct. I can try.

Th. Tell me how high is your guilt compared to when we began on a scale of 1–10? (*Her guilt dropped 4 points. It was a start.*)

Guilt over Setting Boundaries

A parent feels guilt because she sees disappointment on her son's face after telling him that he can't stay out late with his friends. I reflect her conflicted feelings:

Th: That is hard, isn't it? You set the limit because you love your son, and yet you also feel sad knowing that your boundaries disappoint him. What's that like to notice this internal conflict that arises when you set limits with a son you love, knowing you have to disappoint him to be a good parent? (*Helping her to recognize that setting healthy boundaries does not warrant guilt.*)

Absorbing Another's Negative Projections

A woman berates herself when her friend reacts strongly because she forgot her birthday.

Ct: My friend was distraught that I forgot her birthday. How could I have been so thoughtless! It ruined her day.

Th: I've had the same question myself. Could it be that we're universally human? Have you been aware of a harsh voice within yourself that judges you mercilessly? Maybe your friend's deep pain has other roots.

Human limitations will cause us to inevitably disappoint others, no matter how much we try to fix these shortcomings. Sensitivity to others' needs is a worthy but imperfect quest, and I continue to find people's toes beneath my feet despite my best efforts to avoid stepping on them.

A mother described her massive efforts to have spectacular celebrations for her son and daughter. She'd drop everything for them, yet she'd feel like a failure if she saw disappointment or anger in their eyes. Keeping up this pace took a toll on her health and kept her perpetually anxious. I suggested she repeat saying aloud to her son in a fantasy, "There are times I can't do as you wish." Or "I must disappoint you." As she voiced these statements, she became short of breath. I wondered aloud what was she feeling underneath her anxiety and guilt? After some moments of silence, grief gushed out of her as she remembered being a latchkey kid, left alone for extended periods, sitting alone in the darkness and becoming frozen. For the first time, she admitted she hadn't had an idyllic childhood and registered how much pain she'd had as a child. When she realized she was far more available to her son than her mother had been to her, she began to feel less pressured and guilty. She also became less anxious when she explored her feelings toward her mother.

Repressive Defenses against Healthy Guilt

Jon Frederickson (2013) gives examples of repressive defenses against guilt:

Denial ("I didn't mean anything by it.")

Rationalization ("The reason I did it was that you were being a jerk.")

Minimization ("I think you are too sensitive about it.")

Awareness of injurious behavior, compassion, and will to feel healthy remorse

When I hear a defense against guilt, I employ the Healing Triad (Awareness, Compassion, and Will) once more. Some sample interventions would be:

"When you brush off the significance of having hurt your girlfriend, the damage will continue for both you and her. Could we talk about this reality without devaluing you in any way?"

"You may have intended no harm, and she may have been sensitive, but your words still stung. You could lose her if you continually dismiss her feelings. Would you be willing to explore your feelings for having hurt someone you love?"

"I understand why you'd want to shift the focus to your girlfriend (*awareness of defense*). I've hurt people I love too, and it's painful to face. (*Self-disclosure to reduce shame and increase the capacity for guilt*). The reality remains that several people have pulled away from you in similar instances (*awareness of denial*), and we have an opportunity to create something new for you and her. Would you be willing to look at the fact that you're doing something that hurts others?

Healthy Guilt = Remorse and Repair

While self-punishment destroys relationships, healthy remorse heals both partners. Healthy guilt dynamically moves through the body and is proportional to the injury. It distinguishes between:

Unintended harm: e.g., hurting someone due to forgetfulness

Intentional cruelty: e.g., bullying, vandalism, verbal abuse

Unconscious injurious acts: lack of attunement to a child due to depression

A repair for an offense can range from an apology to a long-term, meaningful personal effort. Everyone inflicts pain on those they love, but without the caring to help heal these wounds, we live on the surface of relationships. We'll never experience the fullness of love. When clients avoid repairs, we can explore the cost of these defenses. We can ask:

"How will you feel if you don't express your remorse to your friend?

"If we listen to your guilt about your aunt, what does your guilt say to you?"

"If you avoid making a repair, do you deprive yourself of a valuable relationship?"

"Why would you want to miss an opportunity to heal?"

"Do you want to deny yourself peace of mind and the satisfaction of resolution?"

"Since you've seen that your trauma has passed from your father to your son, what would you want to do with these realizations? Do you think of apologizing to your son?"

It takes courage to face someone and admit our errors. I might share a personal experience when I apologized to someone important and would include helpful details.

Not all Apologies are the Same

Apologies vary in quality significantly. Most apologies are sorely inadequate. A cursory "Sorry" can add salt to a wound. When we make excuses, we dismiss our responsibility and negate the apology. Apologies are best that stand alone. When we start talking about ourselves in the midst of an apology, we defeat the purpose to tend to the injured one. The best apology happens when we step into the other's skin and stay present until we've done all we can to alleviate the other's suffering. Imagine how it feels to endure humiliation, dismissal, broken promises, betrayal, or abandonment. Good apologies aren't rushed. We sit together, make eye contact, express profound regret for the pain we've caused, and leave plenty of space for the wounded other to express anger or pain. There's time for other things later (Shulman, 2017).

Clients often need our guidance with effective apologies, which may be one of the most valuable communication skills we can possess. When death or distance makes it impossible to make amends, the opportunity always exists to apply our guilt lessons in future relationships. When Dennis and Paul could accept their rage and complex feelings and internalize the compassion that I felt toward them, they left their cells of solitary confinement and found their true home, a place where they could love and be loved.

References

Abbass, A. A., & Town, J. M. (2013). Key clinical processes in intensive short-term dynamic psychotherapy. *Psychotherapy, 50*(3), 433–437. https://doi.org/10.1037/a0032166

Abbass, A., Town, J., Ogrodniczuk, J., Joffres, M., & Lilliengren, P. (2017). Intensive short-term dynamic psychotherapy trial therapy: Effectiveness and role of "unlocking the unconscious". *Journal of Nervous and Mental Disease, 205*(6), 453–457. https://doi.org/10.1097/NMD.0000000000000684

Arnold, M. B. (1970). *Feelings and emotions: The Loyola symposium*. Academic Press.

Carveth, D. (2001). The unconscious need for punishment: Expression or evasion of the sense of guilt? *Psychoanalytic Studies*, 9–21. https://doi.org/10.1080/14608950020026827

Damasio, A. R. (2004). Emotions and feelings: A neurobiological perspective. In A. S. R. Manstead, N. Frijda & A. Fischer (Eds.), *Feelings and emotions: The Amsterdam symposium* (pp. 49–57). Cambridge University Press. https://doi.org/10.1017/CBO9780511806582.004

Davanloo, H. (2000). *Intensive short-term dynamic psychotherapy: Selected papers of Habib Davanloo*. Wiley.

Ferguson, T., Stegge, H., & Damhuis, I. (1991). Children's understanding of guilt and shame. *Child Development*, 62(4), 827–839. doi:10.2307/1131180

Frederickson, J. (2013). *Co-creating change: Effective dynamic therapy techniques*. Seven Leaves Press.

Frederickson, J. (2012, April 8). *Guilt: Conscious and Unconscious*. https://istdpinstitute.com/2012/guilt-conscious-and-unconscious/

Izard, C. E. (1978). On the ontogenesis of emotions and emotion-cognition relationships in infancy. In M. Lewis & L. A. Rosenblum (Eds.), *The development of affect* (pp. 389–413). Plenum Press.

Kochanska, G., Gross, J. N., Lin, M. H., & Nichols, K. E. (2002). Guilt in young children: Development, determinants, and relations with a broader system of standards. *Child Development, 73*(2), 461–482. https://doi.org/10.1111/1467-8624.00418

Sroufe, L. (1979). Socioemotional development. In J. Osofsky (Ed.), *Handbook of infant development* (pp. 462–516). Wiley.

Shulman, D. (2017). *ABCs of love: Learn how couples rekindle desire and get happy again*. Shaper House Press.

Tangney, J. P., Stuewig, J., & Mashek, D. J. (2007). Moral emotions and moral behavior. *Annual Review of Psychology, 58*(1), 345–372.

Twelve steps and twelve traditions. (1989). Alcoholics Anonymous World Services.

Warshow, S. (2002). Treatment of a self-defiling, recovering alcoholic with an avoidant personality. *AD HOC Bulletin of Short-Term Dynamic Psychotherapy, 6*(1).

Warshow, S. (2003). Even strangers loved me better. Treatment of a severely fragile, traumatized patient. *AD HOC Bulletin of Short-Term Dynamic Psychotherapy, 7*(1).

9

DISARMING DEFENSES DEFTLY

Ruptures or stalemates often spring up as we're working with entrenched defenses. The way we think and feel about defenses impacts how we respond to them. We may become discouraged, impatient, or angry if we believe a client is walling us out and doesn't budge despite our efforts. Our feelings can intensify when the client becomes argumentative, defiant, or disparaging. In retaliation, the therapist may act out with biting words or thinly disguised contempt. Sometimes we exacerbate trauma. A large body of psychoanalytic and psychodynamic literature published through the 1950's to 1970's addresses destructiveness as it manifests in therapists. (Main, 1957, 1989; Winnicott, 1948). However, if I view these defenses as self-protective strategies used by a vulnerable child to survive, I may feel more compassion and stay engaged. Defenses display the client's history of trauma. Whether responding to fragile, regressive or repressive states (see Figures 9.1 and 9.2), we must reach for a tender place within ourselves to create the safety and attunement for change to occur. As clients become healthier, and the therapeutic relationship feels more secure, the need for defenses decreases. Sometimes, it is not easy for the therapist to move into a compassionate state. Still, we can generate more compassion within us with practice and intention, knowing that self-protective strategies are responses to fears that the therapist will attack, discard, fail,

DOI: 10.4324/9780429399633-10

DEFENSE RECOGNITION
Therapists will find it invaluable to recognize defenses and understand their functions rapidly. Developing this knowledge takes time, experience, and patience with oneself. The less internal pressure we feel, the easier it is to absorb new information and transmit compassion. Caring, clinical intuition, skills, and appropriate timing are necessary to address the defenses with shame sensitivity. There are variations in the categorizations of defenses since Sigmund Freud. These charts offer one useful guide, and they are not all-inclusive.

Figure 9.1 Defense Recognition.

TYPES OF DEFENSES	EXAMPLES (Frederickson, 2013)
TACTICAL DEFENSES: *(Avoid emotional closeness)*	Vagueness, Generalization, Indirect speech, Cover words, Diversification, Retraction, Evasiveness, Distancing
REPRESSIVE DEFENSES: *(Keep feelings out of awareness)*	Intellectualization, Rationalization, Displacement, Minimization, Denial, Reaction formation, Isolation of affect, Avoidance, Instant repression, Identification w/the aggressor, Identification w/the object of one's rage, Suppression
REGRESSIVE DEFENSES: *(Ego functioning regresses)*	Projection, Externalization, Sarcasm, Discharge, Acting out, Defiance, Weepiness, Contempt, Dissociation, Helplessness/Passivity, Somatization

Figure 9.2 Types of Defenses.

or otherwise hurt the client. Probably my greatest challenge has been to remain persistent in working with the client's defenses at times when I've felt like giving up prematurely.

A corporate vice-president presented himself with consummate confidence, charm, and wit. His false self was impenetrable and manipulative. Massive losses finally brought him to AA. But without the bottle, his eyes telegraphed the terror he'd felt as a child when he was brutally beaten by his father in a backyard shed. He found it excruciating to be seen beneath his grandiosity. He had to hide any shortcomings from his father or he could lose his life. Understandably, he was highly resistant to revealing his pain and flaws. The tragedy of alienation from human connection calls for our compassion, the heart of all meaningful defense work.

"A highly resistant patient can use 150 defenses in a fifty-minute session" (Frederickson, 2013, p. 17). We might shudder at this statement, wondering how we can track such rapid, complex phenomena. But as we become increasingly familiar with the defensive strategies, we will recognize them instantly. We ask ourselves, "What is preventing me from feeling closer to this person at this moment?" Our clinical intuition will provide valuable cues. Working skillfully with defenses becomes doable with time and practice. I never met a therapist who hasn't expressed an enormous relief to have an effective orientation to the defenses.

Employ the Healing Triad to Dissolve Defense

Once a vision of the client's hopes for treatment comes into focus, three key elements can ignite momentum and disarm self-protective barriers whenever therapy is stalling.

Awareness of Self-Protective Strategies

Name the barriers to closeness (defenses), so the client can see them:

> "It looked like all the life drains from your body as you enter a state of detachment, where neither of us can find you."
>
> *Mia, a young woman, decided in therapy that she wanted to break the family pattern of talking in superficialities. She took the leap to reveal to her mother and siblings that she'd been in treatment for panic attacks.*

Ct: I told Mom I'd been discovering how much I keep inside me, and I've learned in therapy that this is causing panic attacks. I told her I want to be more open because it's essential for my health.

Th: How did your mother respond?

Ct: She said if I were in therapy, I must be talking about her. Then she said that I was the most shut down of my siblings, and my brother and sister had always been more open than me. Mom said that I'm the most like my dad. (*She smiled without expression covering flashes of feeling.*)

We'd talked a lot about her habit of smiling over her feelings. I began to feel anger at her mother, which Mia disowned. Mia's dad died a couple of years ago. I fantasized that Mia's mom wanted to absolve herself of guilt, hold her husband responsible for Mia's problems, and reassure herself that her other children were fine. She offered no compassion for her daughter's terrible suffering from panic attacks.

Th: How did you feel about your mother's response?

Ct: I felt sadness. Disappointment. (*She said she felt the loss of her father and began to cry. She had no parent to turn to for emotional support.*) It's always about my mother. I had two parents, right? She was involved in how I turned out. (*She had a moment of holding her mother accountable but quickly squashed her angry feelings by describing the tough life her mother had led, rationalizing her emotional absence.*)

Th: You're a compassionate person, and you care for your mother. That's not going to change. But you took a brave step to reveal yourself to your family. I imagine you had feelings when your mother focused on herself and showed little interest in your suffering. You said you were sad and disappointed. Of course you were! Would you want to see how you feel about your mom disappointing you? (*Her next response came down like a judge's gavel. Her voice rose, and she spoke emphatically. Her face was determined and frozen, with a distant smile.*)

Ct: But she won't stop me! She may not like what I told her, but that's too bad. I'm moving on. I've already thought a lot about this, and it's just how it is. (*She began to diversify with other stories and again ignored my question. I felt the force of her resistance, trying to pin me behind her wall. Each therapist must ask, will I be silenced by the defenses or continue to voice my observations? I ask permission.*)

Th: May I reflect on what I'm experiencing at this moment? (*She consented.*) I'm aware that you took a significant risk with your mother, and I've asked a couple of times about your feelings. You came into therapy knowing your feelings are blocked, which affects your marriage and causes panic attacks. You and I agreed we'd give our attention to your feelings in the moment. Your response just then felt like a wall, a strong force telling me to back off. (*I raised my hands like a barricade.*) It was very powerful. What do you experience?

Ct: I notice I'm doing that smiling thing a lot too.

Th: Yes! I'm glad you're aware. What does that tell us?

Ct: I'm doing what I always do. It's familiar. But I have to change this. (*She thought awhile.*) I have to change this for my children. I don't want to pass this on to them, and I know I will if I don't change.

Th: So they won't have panic attacks too? (*Her eyes filled with love and concern, as she agreed. Her children's welfare was a driving motivation. She shifted toward revealing herself.*)

Ct: I felt sad, mad, let down. I thought she'd reach out to me more after my dad died, but she didn't. She's given me no more attention. She just found another guy. She's always been somewhere else.

Th: Tell me about the mad part.

Ct: Oh, I feel mad. I can feel mad. (*She shared that anger was far more familiar to her than she'd ever told me. Anger came out in occasional explosive outbursts with her kids.*)

Th: Where do you feel it?

Ct: All over the place. I feel it everywhere, all the time. (*She gestured throughout her body.*)

Th: I'm glad you're telling me. I didn't know.

Ct: I never discuss anger with my mother.

Th: So you silence this essential part of you with me, as though I'm like your mother. That's very natural in therapy for these old scripts to play out in our relationship. It's good because it gives us a new chance to work with patterns that hurt you.

We began working on her projections that she had to follow the same rules with me that she followed with her Mom. She saw that she couldn't help herself or her kids if she didn't make this effort in therapy. Addressing her wall in this session gave us a chance to talk about her distancing defense so she could become conscious of its origin and her choices today. We'd cleared a path to explore her rage and complex feelings.

Where do we focus first in raising awareness?

When multiple barriers (SAGSS) present themselves, therapists ask, "Where do I focus first?" In a moment we'll talk about Beth, who compulsively talked over my words. Do we address Beth's anxiety, shame, or rapid speech? I don't advocate hard rules, but I ask, "What can the client most easily see?" We don't want to overwhelm the client with too much information. In Beth's case, I began to raise awareness of her racing speech, a self-protective strategy. Anxiety and shame triggered her defense but were outside of her awareness. If we start at the surface, her racing speech, we're in the moment with her. She gets it. She will have to slow down first before she can give attention to her anxiety and shame. We can explore later what lies beneath her rapid speech. The client's response will let us know soon enough what works and what doesn't. Also, when the therapist shares the direct impact of the defenses on their interpersonal relationship, the interaction becomes alive, immediate, and emotionally engaging.

The Therapeutic Transfer of Compassion for Self (TTCS)

The TTCS takes two active partners, both energetically engaged in passing a baton, as we see on an Olympic team. The client will need to be willing, consciously or unconsciously, to receive the transfer of compassion, and the therapist will often have to assist the client in becoming receptive.

When there is resistance to the TTCS, bring it to light:

Th: I feel much caring for your suffering. But I'm not sure that you feel that caring too. My caring won't help you unless you receive it from me and begin directing it toward yourself. To show our mutual caring, we'll want to intervene in any process that isolates you or causes you to disconnect from what you feel. Tell me how this sounds to you? Would you want to direct this kind of compassion toward yourself?

Therapists will need to check their internal state of compassion honestly. Do I feel compassion for this person who has such difficulty sustaining a relationship and pushes me away? The defenses invite us to disengage, the path of least resistance. Are we pulling back or shutting down? Are we lounging in our chair or getting tired? Is our vocal tone flat? Are we talking without feeling? We are unlikely to help a client become freer from defenses if we are in a defensive state ourselves. Our compassionate words will have little effect if the client doesn't have an embodied experience of our caring. An alternative is to dig deep and say with feeling:

Th: I feel great concern for your future and the possibility that you will remain lonely. Yet, I can do nothing to change this tragic course if you do not care as I do. I will remain sad for a long time, but your sadness will last many more years, and that's such a painful reality.

Or:

Th: You've said you're willing for us to give attention to your feelings. I believe feelings just came up in you, but when I show caring interest in them, you become argumentative and it feels like a wall between us. My compassion will mean nothing if we're not in this together. I want to respect your wishes, so please let me know where we go from here.

The Will

The "will" or "intention" (Dyer, 2014) to feel and relate is a subtle yet amazing force that becomes activated when we care for ourselves. When we care, we won't watch from the sidelines when we see self-harming forces wreak damage in our lives. In this following case, I hope to mobilize the client's will to intervene on her behalf.

Engaging the will to refrain from talking over the therapist

Beth's compulsive, racing speech leaves others far behind. Her pressured speech blankets the anxiety, shame, and other feelings that lie beneath her defenses. Such patterns often continue for months or years in session. If the therapist never brings this pattern to Beth's attention, what happens? Even if the therapist manages to reduce her anxiety in specific situations, her unconscious habit of "talking over" other people will continue to damage her relationships. She won't recognize other people's responses, and she'll remain unaware of her body signals *and feelings, blocking emotional closeness. Imagine using a tender tone of voice and embodied compassion in this exchange with Beth, who was ruminating about a date:*

Th: I'm sorry for your disappointment with your date. You've thought a lot about the unfortunate experiences you've had with men. You're a very astute woman, and I think you've come to see me because you seek something outside your awareness to stop this pattern of suffering. (*She nods yes.*) But I get the sense that you feel so much internal pressure that your words come fast, and they leave little space for either of us to respond deeply. It's like you won't have enough time to get everything out. Or perhaps you have so much feeling inside that it feels overwhelming? Tell me how it seems to you. Do you see what I mean? (*Said softly, caringly.*)

Ct: Yes. I want to be sure I cover everything. I'm always racing. Sorry to interrupt. (*She looks down in shame.*)

Th: I fully accept you as you are, Beth. I, too, want us to cover all that is important for you. Noticing your internal experience also feels crucial, so you can tap into the value of your feelings and get something new from our relationship. It's a shame for you to live with this pressure, which I imagine is related to anxiety about revealing yourself to me in this vulnerable way. I wonder if we might attempt to go slower so we can both process the experiences you're describing?

Ct: You're not the first person who has said something about this to me. I have a lot of fears about time passing by, and wondering why have I failed in relationships?

Th: Perhaps if we slow down and help you to feel less anxious, you'll be more able to connect to others.

She saw how she'd been cutting off my sentences and felt some momentary shame, a healthy response. Her new awareness caused her to slow down her rapid speech, and she saw that her self-absorbed date was not the only one dismissing her feelings. She cried as she saw the price of her defense, which left her no way to tune in to herself or anyone else. If I had withheld my observations, Beth would have kept talking over herself and me, and her therapy would be less productive.

She believed she was very close to her children and her friends, and of course, they loved each other. But when she talks compulsively, much is lost, including listening, sharing silence together, and inquiring into each other's feelings. Many clients have no idea how they keep others at a distance, but when they recognize the damage caused by their defenses, they have both grief and excitement for an opportunity for a new life.

Principles of *Shame Sensitive* Defense Work

Raising awareness of self-protective strategies and making way for underlying feelings is potentially life changing, but implementation can present a minefield. The client may feel criticized as we draw attention to problematic patterns and react by becoming less accessible. Using *shame sensitive* principles while addressing defenses (as well as toxic shame, anxiety and guilt), reduces the perception of disapproval and raises hope. *Shame sensitivity* is not the same as shame avoidance. Instead, it recognizes and responds compassionately to shame states. Shame reactions often accompany new awareness of self-harming intrapersonal processes. Here are a few of the defining elements of *shame-sensitivity*:

1. Gain permission to address defenses and respect the client's choice
2. Explore defensive process collaboratively
3. Attune to the vulnerability of releasing defenses
4. Seek to transfer compassion for the cost of defenses
5. Never imply judgment for the defenses
6. Use vivid language that evokes compassion for the cost of defenses
7. Empathize with the conflict to relinquish defenses
8. Clarify the path to overcome defenses and point out successes
9. Normalize defenses as a resourceful responses to trauma
10. Always offer a clear alternative to a defense
11. Separate the person from the defenses
12. Self-disclose our personal struggles with defenses
13. Explore cultural influences on defenses

Gain Permission to Address Defenses and Respect the Client's Choice

It is the client's choice to discuss their defenses and reveal their inner experience to the therapist. We can assume the client's will aligns with ours, but we have no way of knowing this until it's made explicit (e.g., "I no longer want to fear my feelings, and I want to stop pushing people away.") The alliance is also expressed implicitly (e.g., the client reveals a hidden, painful memory). Permission to address the defenses is part of a collaborative alliance. Assuming we have an agreement to reveal feelings and body sensations, we might say, "I know you want more access to your feelings. Your feelings know how to feel, but they've been discouraged. Is it ok if we talk about anything that would prevent you from accessing them? If we join forces to move the barriers out of the way, your feelings will find freedom. Does this make sense for you?"

It's tempting to press a client toward releasing feelings without checking on the client's will. The therapist's shame or strong desire to get results can cause us to pressure the resistance in a way the client may perceive as dominating or intimidating, leading to compliance, a weak alliance, or defiance. The desire to overcome defenses must come from within the client, not only the therapist.

Explore Defensive Process Collaboratively (The Sherpa Therapist)

Our protective barriers belong to us, and it is no one's right to wrench them from us. When we help our clients to discover their defenses, many recognize their impact and draw insightful conclusions with little help. If we are to have a respectful, equal relationship, all explorations require the client's choice. Schore said (2012), "...respect for the individual is, and always has been, paramount." In this spirit, the therapist is like a Sherpa. The Sherpa guides the climber who wishes to reach a particular summit. The Sherpa does not push, pull, persuade, or coerce. He simply points the way for a safe and successful climb, offering a steady, caring presence. But sometimes, the therapist's desires for success overtake the client's will, creating the impression that we expect something from the client.

Projection of Will

Sometimes the client projects that the therapist wants something rather than the other way around. We call this projection of will. We can remind the client of the reality: the client seeks and the therapist serves, according to the client's will and choice.

In the following vignette, the therapist brings the projection of will to the client's awareness:

Ct: You try to get people to talk about feelings, but there's no evidence that it works (*the client came to therapy to be understood and helped*).

Th: I know it looks like I have an agenda. Of course, I encourage you to express yourself, so that I can help you. But it's essential to respect your choice every step of the way. I don't want to go anywhere without your consent and permission.

This client expects to be abandoned and misunderstood, which gives her a rationale to keep me at a distance. We might be tempted to try to talk her out of her defense, which would invite more resistance and does not stay true to the spirit of collaboration.

Ct: I never feel understood by anyone in my life.

Th: I can only imagine how painful and lonely your experience has been, beginning in your early years. It sounds like you don't expect me to understand either.

Ct: No one has.

Th: What if I didn't understand?

Ct: Then maybe I wouldn't get the help I need.

Th: And how sad that would be! Wouldn't your expectation of not getting enough from me keep you from revealing yourself? I'm sure we'd have to go back and forth to arrive at an understanding at times, but I am motivated to do my best. But I wouldn't be perfect, and you would have feelings along the way. What do you imagine feeling in those moments when I may not understand you?

Ct: Frustration. Maybe disappointment. (*Frustration and disappointment are secondary feelings. They both trigger primary feelings.*)

Th: Your desire to be understood would be frustrated, right? And that's certainly not what you would want. So your desires would be disappointed and frustrated.

Ct: Yeah.

Th: And then what would you feel?

Ct: If you didn't understand me, I'd feel alone.

Th: You'd feel alone, like I had abandoned you. And then what do you feel? (*Abandonment is a state that is attached to feelings. Return to focus on feelings.*)

Ct: Then I'm—that's probably a comfortable place—alone with my sadness. I'm more comfortable alone.

Th: So then you would put up a wall?

Ct: Yeah, because it's never done any good to let anybody in.

Th: Yeah. And then what does the wall do? (*What is the cost of defense?*)

Ct: It prevents connection.

Th: Yes. And how tragic is that? You grew up without the possibility of connection, and so you protected yourself with a wall. You gave up trying to connect. I would do the same thing. But now, the wall perpetuates the loneliness of your childhood, causing immeasurable suffering. The wall seals you off. And what does it do for your desire to help you trust yourself and know yourself?

Ct: None of it will happen.

Th: It's just very sad. I understand your desire to stay in a cocoon, and of course you can. But another part of you came here for something more fulfilling, and I'd love to support your deepest desires. But your choice will determine our direction (*hoping to raise her awareness that we each have a role in a positive outcome*).

Attune to the Vulnerability of Releasing Defenses

When we introduce our clients to their defenses and the feelings that lie beneath them, they may feel confused, criticized, or inadequate. Even asking what clients feel can evoke shame because they do not recognize their emotional states. Even though sensations occur in our bodies all the time, few clients pay attention to them or relate them to their emotions. Being attuned to the vulnerability of recognizing and releasing defenses is crucial to creating safety in the relationship.

In the following vignette, a woman shows confusion about identifying her feelings. While confusion is a defense, I prefer not to point out her confusion as in, "You become confused as we begin to explore your feelings." I begin with the assumption that confusion calls for further clarification and assistance, such as:

Ct: I had an unpleasant talk with my ex yesterday. He expects me to change our schedules with the children all the time.

Th: How are you feeling toward him?

Ct: I don't know what you're looking for when you ask me how I feel. I'm not good at feelings. I really don't understand. (*The client feels inadequate to identify her feelings and fears displeasing the therapist.*)

Th: Many people have trouble identifying feelings. (*Normalizing her confusion to reduce shame.*) You're not alone. If it's ok with you (*seeking permission and offering an alternative*), you might try a simple body scan to see if you notice any sensations. If you don't notice anything, that's helpful to know too. There is no right or wrong response, and the more we can relieve any performance pressure, the better. (*She will be less able to identify her feelings when her shame is high.*) Even small body signals give us cues to what you're feeling. (*Some who cannot name their emotions are often able to identify sensations in the body through focusing.*)

Ct: I think there's some heat in my mid-section. Some tightness in my shoulders.

Th: Oh, that's great! You notice some heat and muscle activation as you tell me about your ex-husband. (*A focus on a specific person and recent event help people to connect to feelings.*) Do you sense any emotion accompanying the heat and shoulder tightness?

Ct: Annoyance. (*Progress toward identifying her angry feelings. I begin to track the client's comprehension as I link her body sensations to feelings toward her ex.*)

Th: The heat in your mid-section tells us that annoyance and related feelings became activated about your ex-husband, which is so natural. We see you're able to identify feelings, which is great. The muscle tension suggests a tightening around your emotions. Your confusion about what you feel is part of a system to discourage you from exploring your feelings. Does this make sense for you? Please tell me how you understand what I'm saying. (*Allowing space for her to reflect is crucial. It's new for her to realize that confusion restricts an exploration of her feelings and that her body sensations can help us identify them.*)

Ct: I guess I'm wondering why I'd want to stay away from my feelings. But definitely, I ignore them. That's a pretty new idea to realize my body provides some cues.

Seek to Transfer Compassion for the Cost of Defenses

The therapist's authentic, body-based compassion for the horrific suffering caused by defenses helps our clients feel safer with us and more likely to feel compassion for themselves. Schore (2012) stresses the importance of being present with the client, especially during stressful times, and states, "An attachment based clinical approach highlights the unconscious nonverbal affective factors more than conscious verbal cognitive factors as the essential change process of psychotherapy." Raising awareness of maladaptive, dysfunctional defenses triggers shame and resistance, which can frustrate the therapist. It can be tough to feel compassion while a defense is defeating the therapy. So we may have to work with ourselves before we work with our clients. When we shift into a state of compassion, our acceptance and caring will be transmitted through our choice of words, vocal tone, body language, and eye gaze, which evoke self-caring in the client. Self-compassion replaces the shame triggered by defense work.

A severely depressed woman said upon termination:

"Your face comes to mind so often when I am in one of my moods where I'm unkind to myself, and a voice comes up that says, "Be gentle with yourself. I see your eyes, and I see the compassion that comes from them, and I "remember" to be present and real in my gentleness, to stop the self-hatred and stop the sabotaging personality from making me miserable."

Samples of verbalizing compassion for the cost of various defenses

Vagueness: "How very sad that it is unfamiliar to declare or define what you want."

Minimization: "Your desires for yourself seem so meager. It's terrible you've had to adapt to so much deprivation."

Denial of desire: "What a shame that your needs had to hide in the shadows like they have no importance or right to exist at all."

Storytelling, an intellectualizing defense

An exchange with a client who starts in storytelling mode and my attempts to help her move toward her feelings:

Ct: I've been feeling pretty down. My husband blew up at me the other day. He cursed and told me how ridiculous I am for asking him to try to be quieter while I was talking on the phone to my sister. He was making a lot of noise with our dogs. He didn't see why this was such a big deal and said I'm way too critical. Then he just left the house and didn't say goodbye. Then my girlfriend called me and began telling me about her latest cooking class and she ran into our mutual friend, Gloria. I've never particularly cared for Gloria...

Th: May I interrupt a moment? You must feel very painful emotions about your husband devaluing you and then walking out. I'm noticing that your mind moves to other thoughts and memories, which seems unfortunate because your important feelings are left in the dust. Going into a thinking mode has probably been a way to move away from your pain, but so much of you is left behind. (*Separating feeling from defense and seeking to raise compassion*).

Rationalizing, self-blame:

Ct: Well, he has a point. I probably had a tone in my voice. I just start feeling stupid, like, "Why did I do that?" I could certainly have managed to talk to my sister without having to interrupt his fun. He works hard, and he's right that his home should be a place to relax.

Th: I'm sure that both of you have legitimate needs and desires. But I wonder where your feelings go? Frankly, I feel sad that they are so quickly dismissed.

Rationalization and turning feelings of anger against the self:

Ct: (*Lowering head*). It just seems selfish or like it shouldn't be necessary. I think I could adapt more, be less needy, and more cooperative.

Th: You place importance on your husband's reaction, yet your feelings remain off the radar, not even a consideration.

Ct: It just seems normal. Guess I've been off the radar for most of my life. (*Sighs with sadness.*)

Inviting compassion toward herself:

Th: I sense your pain, and I surely feel it for you. If your daughter came home distressed after someone had bullied her in the play yard, would you be likely to ignore her fear or her tears? Would you say that the bully had a rough day?

Ct: No, of course not. I would never ignore her like that. She's everything to me. I'd go to her. I'd hold her. I'd tell her I love her. I might even report the person who did that to her.

Th: You would go to great lengths to care for her, but for some reason, you are not worthy of the same kind of attention? What you described as selfish, I describe as self-care. For some reason, this is not something you expect for yourself?

Ct: No. My father used to lock me out of the house when I cried. I felt like a pathetic, despicable person. I felt wrong to be such a burden to him.

Th: How horrific for you! I feel such sadness for what you endured. Might we extend some compassion to you for having been shunned at your most vulnerable moments? Your father taught you to treat yourself with indifference to your pain. How does that feel for us to look at this?

Ct: It makes me sad.

Th: Please allow yourself to feel this sadness. This sadness is an expression of caring and compassion for yourself. (*She cries. I ask how it feels to share this sadness with me.*)

Ct: It feels good to be able to cry. I don't think I've ever done this before in front of someone.

Th: It feels good to me that you share your sadness with me. I appreciate you're letting me in. Tell me how you experience my response to this grief inside you.

Ct: I see that you care.

Th: Indeed, I do.

Never Imply Judgment for the Defenses

Every nuance of our communication, including phraseology, intonation, and body language, sends a message while we're working with defenses. I've mentioned that I attempt to avoid "you messages," especially when talking about defenses. Although all of us use this language and it can work, still, when we say "You are attacking yourself" or "You are avoiding your feelings," we risk inviting shame. Communications experts advise us to avoid "you messages" because they are likely to make people defensive and imply intent (Bippus & Young, 2005; Gordon, 1975; Gottman & Silver, 1999). Which "you" are we talking about?

In an interview with David Bullard, Allan Schore commented:

> Most of my ideas about the self-come from neuroscience and psychoanalysis, including Jung and others. But the idea of self/nonself and multiple self states have been a focus. In current relational psychoanalytic writings the concept that comes closest to my own is Philip Bromberg's idea about multiplicity of self-states: that we all have a variety of self states associated with different affects and motivations. Some of these are operating on a conscious level, others of these on unconscious levels. He calls these latter states "not-me" states as opposed to "me" states (a concept he borrowed from Harry Stack Sullivan).
>
> (Bullard, 2015)

While defenses are seen as part of the self, "That's just who I am," they are formed unconsciously and outside our will and volition. Since people tend to be defensive about their defenses, and defenses are mostly unconscious, I don't want to imply the client is purposely using defenses. I prefer talking about them as operations, systems, or forces that victimize my client. Once defenses become conscious, our clients can begin to exercise choices. But this is not easy, and we always want to convey empathy for the unconscious grip of defenses, once necessary for survival, and the damage they create.

Sometimes substituting one word or phrase or a shift in inflection radically changes how our words land. I can convey pathos or a hard challenge with the same comment. "I can only imagine the trauma that caused you to become so suspicious of other people *(said tenderly)*" vs. "It seems you don't trust me" and you've put up a wall *(with an edge in my voice)*.

In this next vignette, I am framing the client's defenses as learned, automatic, and unconscious. Kristen was frantic about her inability to hold onto a partner and disturbed by her mother's estrangement. She often asked my opinion about something she'd read, enticing me to engage with her intellectually. I resisted, not wanting to collude with her hurtful intellectualizing habits.

Th: Kristen, if I answer your questions, we'll sadly be taking a detour away from your feelings. You've spent years in therapy seeking this type of understanding. Perhaps you've had unfortunate experiences that have conditioned you outside of your awareness to rely on your intellect at the expense of your feelings. (*As opposed to, "You are intellectualizing."*) Has it brought you relief from your suffering?

Ct: No, not really. But please, please, this is really important, and you'll see how it relates to what I'm trying to explain. (*"Explain" introduces another intellectualization.*) Honestly—

Th: We can go down that road, but I don't think it will help you. I fear that our time will run out, and I'm sad that your excruciating pain and sense of aloneness will continue. (*The therapist often must withstand internal pressure to respond helpfully. I couldn't stop her from saying what she wanted to say, but I could at least give her my compassionate perspective.*)

Ct: Ok. Well, I'm not happy with the way my boyfriend takes sides with my parents. He doesn't respect me. He makes me angry. (*She shifted and showed a welcome interest in herself, yet her physiological responses—tears and agitation—did not match the neurobiological expression of anger.*)

Th: I'm so glad you could tell me of your anger. You're able to recognize what you feel in a cognitive sense (*isolation of affect*). Would you also want to give attention to your body and see how your anger feels?

Ct: I know what I feel! (*Said insistently.*)

She launched into an argument that there was nothing more to discover about her emotions, and a torrent of words followed, pulling both of us downriver. I found footing by simply saying:

Th: You've told me you'd tried many approaches and still feel stuck. When I suggest we focus on your feelings, which exist in your body, you explain how you see this differently. I'm glad you express your perspective, but I wonder if these views are working for you? (*Tone of voice will determine if my question sounds challenging, sincere, caring, respectful, or rhetorical? I invite her to reflect on the impact of her stance with softness.*)

Ct: Whatever I'm doing is not working (*said with sadness*). I'm still stuck. What would I be doing differently if I were to feel my emotions? I'd like you to walk me through the process. (*She revealed humility and vulnerability that hadn't been present before. She was unaware that learned habits blocked her natural ability to feel.*)

Th: Just to be clear, it's good you're able to identify the anger you feel toward your boyfriend. Let me try to add to your understanding. Your tears tell us of your pain and sense of powerlessness, but your tears are different from your anger. You lash out with words, but these outbursts don't tell us what the energy of your anger feels like in your body. When your puppies run to you, you know how the impulse to hug them feels in your arms. Right? (*She agrees.*) But you have difficulty feeling your anger. Does it make sense to you that it's important to feel all your emotions as they exist in your body?

Ct: I don't know, but I do see that I need to find a way out of my depression. (*She cries and acknowledges her intense pain over the losses over the last several years.*) I'd like you to guide me.

Th: I'm happy to help, and your willingness to try something new is hopeful. (*Timing becomes crucial here. If we do not recognize that an active alliance has come online, our hesitation to move toward feelings can miss an opportunity.*) Would you tell me about a specific exchange that triggered your anger? (*A time, place and specific details help to stir emotions. She unconsciously diverted from my question numerous times. It's my task to raise her awareness of her avoidant protective strategy.*)

Ct: It was similar to when my sister and me—

Th: We won't be able to explore feelings about several people and multiple occasions at one time. (*Without tenacity in working with defenses, nothing new would likely emerge.*) I notice that each time we explore your feelings toward your boyfriend, **something pulls you in another direction, abandoning your feelings.** (*She is a victim of her defenses.*) I'm concerned you won't have relief by the end of the session, and I care about you. (*Raising awareness of the cost of her diversification.*)

Ct: Ok. What do I feel toward him? (*Silence ensued as she started tracking her bodily sensations.*) The feeling is intense all over my body. I feel explosive! (*A volcanic feeling erupted through her musculature. At the end of the session, she recognized that her tears covered her anger. She saw that her criticisms pushed her boyfriend *away from her, punishing him and her. She ended the session with wonderment in her voice.)*

Ct: Ahh, this has been a revelation! I *never* understood *this* before.

Th: How wonderful! Tell me more about what feels new to you?

Ct: I don't have to behave badly when I'm angry. I've believed that I'm emotionally stunted for decades, but I'm not doomed to enact my parent's behavior when I'm angry. My anger doesn't have to threaten me or anyone else.

Th: How does it feel to come to this realization?

Ct: It feels really cool. I'm less afraid. Amazing! I plan to pay attention in the coming week when I get angry and not say anything I'll regret. I'll try to notice how my anger feels. (*When we persist in the face of defenses, sometimes we find the person behind them. And it's wonderful.*)

Use Vivid Language to Evoke Compassion for the Cost of Defenses

When it comes to defenses, we name them to tame them. When our language is vivid and symbolic, it can become even more impactful and memorable. A woman in mid-life felt despair after years of failed romantic relationships and unquenchable yearnings. She was a colorful storyteller, and she painted the scene of her magical night with a guy she'd met at a dance club, who never called her again. When I asked how she felt toward him, she had severe shortness of breath. I said she had a "boa" tightening its serpent body around her throat, determined to suffocate her rightful feelings. I shared my hunch that this reptile had silenced her for years, leaving her defenseless and powerless to protect herself.

In the second session, as she filled the room with another story, I was quiet while I searched for an organic and non-shaming way to raise her awareness that her Boa was again talking over her feelings. She surprised me by preempting my thoughts, "I'm talking a lot and not revealing anything. Wow! This is an incredible moment! You got me to see something that no one has ever brought up before."

I also sensed that she had complex feelings and asked if she was aware of any other feelings toward me? Her response was fierce and final. She had no feelings, nothing further to say. My questions would go nowhere! It was as if a vacuum had sucked the air out of the room. She told me later that her internal response was, "Back off, sister!" I addressed this fierce wall as something that kept her feeling lonely and separate from others. She left the session tearful, saying she wanted to defeat the Boa and hoped it wasn't bigger than she was. I assured her that together we could overcome it. She and her mother were extremely close, and individuating from her was very threatening. She emailed me later about her fury at her "Boa," which we discovered represented her mother, who shut down her feelings.

Ct: Though I wasn't able to access my feelings at those particular moments during our time together on the way home, it was such another story. I found myself yelling, speaking loudly, I would say. I was crying and yelling at the Boa, and saying 'No more Boa, no more, just no more.' It was very emotional. It was very heave-hoey. As it was happening, I was so grateful to be expressing and emoting. And then I called my brother, and it was beautiful, and it sparked even more tears on the way home. (*She had been distant from her brother.*) And then I came home (*she was in the process of moving*) and I'm still in a purge process before packing. I went through more pictures and just memories and letters people have written me and people whose lives I've touched and never really realized at the time. I just glided through pictures and memories. (*Since she could see her suffocating, devaluing defenses, she was able to separate herself from them and allow herself to take in the love that people had expressed to her over the years.*)

She went on to say:

Ct: It was a very emotional day, and though it may seem that nothing happened during the last session, I took something home with me, and I appreciate it, and I appreciate you. My goal is to trust you and show you these feelings I have in a real, real way. Thank you, and I appreciate you, and I appreciate your way, and I dig it. It is uncharted territory for me, your method, it is new, and so I appreciate your patience.

It was very moving to see how much emotional freedom and self-care she could access from a session in which her wall had so fiercely separated us. Naming her wall (or Boa) allowed her to recognize it, which instilled hope. She saw that she could help our team by paying more attention to her body and resisting her intellectualizing habits.

"The creation of hope is of crucial importance … a central ingredient in overcoming discouragement and producing change" (Greenberg & Paivio, 1997).

Empathize with the Conflict to Relinquish Defenses

The following exchange occurred after I'd drawn attention to a woman's detached body language. She had folded her arms tightly across her chest, and hardened her face. I attempted to explore her internal conflict with her distancing mechanisms.

Detachment

Th: I know you want closer relationships with your women friends, and we could begin with our relationship. I'm noticing your folded arms and sense there is a part of you that wants to distance from me.

Ct: Yes. There's a part that says, "Of course I want to open up." I hadn't been aware that my body says, "No, not at all! Not at any cost!"

Th: Thank you for telling me about your intense conflict. It must be challenging to feel torn between the part of you that wants us to delve into your feelings and this other dominant part that wants you to stay distant (*she nods in agreement*). And I would never want to disrespect you by trying to push through those protective walls (*honoring her choice*), as they're trying to keep you safe. (*Ct: Yeah.*) And only you can know what feels right for you.

Ct: I was totally hostile. I felt, "Don't come too close." (*She makes a hand gesture of pushing me. Any of us might feel rejected, but the client's openness indicates an active therapeutic alliance. The alliance can be high even though resistance is high.*)

Th: Exactly.

Ct: Or I will kill you, or something like this.

Th: So you have these powerful feelings that want to defend you from me, but because you don't feel safe with me, a barrier stops you from expressing those feelings.

Ct: Yeah. That's right.

Th: And what do we do? What do you want us to do about the barrier? (*Engaging with her collaboratively since decisions about defenses belong to her.*)

Ct: I would like this barrier to no longer be there.

Th: You want the freedom to be you and the option for closer relationships. How wonderful! Would you let us help you by taking a look at what you're feeling toward me? Right now? (*Providing an immediate alternative to distancing.*)

Ct: Yeah, we can do it. (*She agrees to explore her feelings but is this compliance? Her answer was quick.*)

Th: Are you saying you're ready to look at your feelings toward me? (*Checking to be sure.*)

Ct: Yes. In a way, you are like an enemy who wants to come way too close to me. (*By identifying me as a perceived enemy, she signals that she would not be ready to reveal herself to me.*)

Th: And it must be quite terrifying to think that I might invade you. (*My next comments remind her of what she wanted from therapy. Only her desire will propel risk-taking.*) Would you agree that there is a part of you who has *asked* me to come close to you so that you might be able to have closer relationships with your female friends? (*She says yes.*) You wanted help with your fear of women and wanted to stop attacking people to protect yourself? You also mentioned that you had back and shoulder tension and wanted to express yourself without fear, is that right? (*She nods affirmatively.*)

Ct: Umm. I want closeness with me but not with you. (*She recognizes the dichotomy within her.*)

Th: Interesting. How do we do this? (She *chuckles*). How do I help you get closer to yourself and be around women without fear when fear dominates our relationship? How do we help you with your distrust of others if you don't take a risk with me, as difficult as it seems? (*Again, seeking her collaboration.*)

Ct: (*Silence for several moments*). Yes, but couldn't we do this without getting into a relationship? So I would like to feel my feelings, but I don't want to express them to you.

Th: Humm. Humm (*empathic*). I honor and respect your right to have a complete choice about this. I care about your well-being, but I have no desire to push you in any direction you don't want to go.

Ct: The truth is that I look forward to our sessions. I love them. I'm not afraid of them. I'm waiting. "Oh, today, I have a session, I like them". (*She takes a significant step in disclosing that I am important to her, despite her attempts to push me away.*)

Th: That's so great. (*Client laughs at the contradiction.*) I wouldn't have thought that from what you said at the beginning. But it's great you're expressing it.

Ct: Yeah, it's different parts inside of me. (*Once she can see her internal conflict, she can make a conscious choice rather than becoming paralyzed by unconscious conflict. She had full breakthroughs toward me and her mother in her therapy and emerged with a remarkably stronger sense of herself.*)

Clarify the Path to Overcome Defenses and Point Out Successes

We increase the client's sense that "I can relinquish my defenses!" when we show faith in the client's capacity, clarify the client's role in our partnership, highlight successes, and reassure our clients that we stand alongside them. When therapists overwork, we usurp the client's role and implicitly underestimate our client's capacity. We also exhaust ourselves.

The Client's Role

As discussed in Chapter 4, both partners have a role to play to move the ball down the court, and we can only score points as a team. Our clients need to understand how they can help themselves. The choice to take risks for health belongs to the client. However, the client can't embark on a journey or choose if he doesn't understand what it entails. Clarifying the road to success is the therapist's responsibility. Should the client agree to this partnership, rich rewards can await.

When appropriate, clarify to the client that the success of therapy will rely upon the client's engagement in the following ways:

A The client's will to explore deeply felt personal goals, the engine of treatment. For many people, revealing what they want triggers shame, so they hide their desires and dreams. I don't take a step forward until we can overcome these barriers. Otherwise, whose goals would we be pursuing?

B The choice to observe and share internal processes (bodily sensations, thoughts, emotions, and perceptions of the relationship) to the best of one's ability. Perfection is not needed ... just the willingness to try.

C The willingness to recognize that shame, anxiety, guilt, and self-protective strategies (SAGSS) cause significant pain in the client's life, defeating one's dreams.

D The desire to pay attention to SAGSS in partnership with the therapist.

E The will to free oneself from SAGSS to tap into one's emotions and desires.

An example of clarifying the client's role and activating the *will to release the defenses of depression and repression:*

Ct: I have no choice when I wake up and feel despair.

Th: If it's true that you have no choice, then we are doomed, but I don't believe that's true. You demonstrate the ability to observe your depressive thoughts, a capacity within you that is separate from your despairing beliefs. Your depressed state did not drive you to my office. As a team, you and I could help you distance yourself from your transient, discouraging thoughts and begin to look at what you feel under your depression instead (*offering an alternative to defense*). You do have a choice, route A or B. That choice is yours to make. (*At first, she had seemed utterly helpless, but after my comments, she shook off her tears and rage rose toward her mother, who had demanded subservience and abandoned her. When we reflected on this session, she was stunned to discover the cruelty of her repression, resulting from a harsh and unfair judgment of her feelings.*)

Normalize Defenses as a Resourceful Responses to Trauma

When we provide context by explaining how defenses warded off trauma, we normalize these protective mechanisms and evoke compassion rather than self-condemnation. For example, "How tragic that your violent father taught you to crush your life force, a habit that now cuts you off from your son. Yet you want to be close to him. Shall we join forces to help you out of this trap?"

Taking the voice of repressed rage to evoke compassion

One woman's profound shame around her slightest aggressive impulse bogged down our work. I tried to give her a sense of the nobility of her abandoned rage, which stemmed from growing up in a culture and family that infantilized and degraded females. I helped to arouse her sympathy for her anger, which protested against repetitive humiliations.

Th: Would you mind if I took the voice of the lioness inside you? (*She gave permission, and I proceeded.*) Why won't you let me out of my cage? What have I done to deserve this cruelty?

Ct: I don't know what you're capable of doing. I have some ugly images when I think about it. (*She recalls instances when family members were explosive.*)

Th: I understand your fears. But you do not lose control as your family did. I'm energy inside you with impulses to protect you, and I could be a great friend to you if you'd allow me. I'm a force of nature, like the wind. I despise being imprisoned for a crime I never committed.

As I took the voice of her anger, I felt strong compassion for her caged feelings. In response, she grew increasingly willing to explore her primitive impulses. She felt a powerful energy in her jaws as her inner lioness fought back and overcame the mother who had belittled her all her life. She felt triumphant and liberated afterward and expressed gratitude for the work we'd been able to achieve.

Always Offer a Clear Alternative to a Defense

A therapist told me he'd felt emotionally bludgeoned by a client, who had enacted an emotionally abusive pattern with him that had obliterated many relationships, causing the client to rely on drugs and live in isolation. She rebuked Steve, her therapist, as incompetent and accused him of being a shill for his agency. Though he was fuming, Steve became anxious and tried to appease her. I suggested he give himself time to feel, reflect, and breathe. If necessary, he could let the client know that he needed a time out to process what just happened. We don't have to respond immediately. We can wait until a genuine response comes to us. Better to be silent than saying something we'll regret.

I encouraged Steve to remember his value. I recall formal lectures where the speakers presented cases in which they'd sat silently listening to torrents of verbal abuse for years. But abuse helps no one. And many clients with severe personality disorders have told me how much they'd learned when I set boundaries on abuse. Everyone deserves respect and kindness, including the therapist. I've witnessed many turning points in treatment when clients recognized I wouldn't be passive while they harmed themselves or me.

In the spirit of authenticity, Steve might say:

Th: I see you're having strong feelings toward me that would be valuable to explore. At the same time, this accusatory way of expressing your emotions makes it harder for me to stay with you. I'm experiencing some of the vulnerability you felt when your mom chastised you relentlessly.

Ct: Well, that's your problem.

Th: Perhaps it is. But when I have a problem, doesn't that affect our relationship? Don't we both lose something? That saddens me, and it concerns me for you. I remember that your mom was indifferent to your feelings, which caused you not to want to be around her. When you've been indifferent to other people's feelings, you've paid a terrible price. If you hold on to the view that I have no value to you or push me away from you, as has happened with other therapists, what happens to the relief you hope to have from our work?

Ct: I know I can't keep living like this.

Th: Then would you want us to pull together as partners and keep an eye on this distancing mechanism and prevent it from eliminating everyone who tries to help you or get close to you?

The therapist offers the client the alternative to use the therapeutic partnership to bring these destructive forces to conscious awareness and push back against them. The therapist will be powerless alone. The client has a choice. She can engage in a mutual effort to restrain her acting out and explore her angry impulses instead.

Another possible response:

Th: Would you agree that the judging part of your mind has distanced you from many people, creating distrust and leaving you

> with feelings of unbearable aloneness? (*Allow moments of silence for reflection.*) Would you agree this pattern is sadly happening between us? Would you want to find a way out of this pattern?

Separate the Person from the Defenses

Drawing attention to the defenses is delicate because our clients are attached to their self-protective strategies. They identify with their defenses and rely upon them. We hope to facilitate a gradual withdrawal from the dependency on defenses, but such an act will trigger every siren behind the prison walls. We need to speak to the part of the self that operates outside the defensive system, namely the wise observer who can recognize the child's trauma, the need and purpose for defense development, the current cost of defenses, and the possibilities beyond the defenses.

Engage the observer

> "Your truest self can observe your detachment. Could we speak to that part of you who can observe your detachment? We both know why you built these walls, yet you long for freedom on the other side."
>
> "How old is that part of you who learned to hide from people?" Is there anything you'd want to say to that part of you?

Self-Disclose Our Struggles with Defenses

We can reduce the client's shame with reminders that difficulties with self-protective patterns are universal and human. I shared a story with a man who struggled to access his anger. I told him I used to be very shy and avoided revealing angry feelings for years. It was a big moment when I first told a friend that I'd felt hurt and disappointed when she'd been unavailable in a crisis. I did not become aggressive, but I expressed my hurt. My client showed surprise that I'd had similar struggles. He exhaled, and his facial muscles relaxed. He thought he was irreparably damaged, but my story helped him to see our shared vulnerability. He also saw how both of us could step outside our protective walls. My disclosure led to the first significant breakthrough to complex feelings in our work.

Explore Cultural Influences on Defenses

We cannot be fully sensitive to shame and defenses if we do not attune to cultural differences and inequities. If these issues go unrecognized, our clients may view us as avoidant, shaming, and disconnected. These significant conversations should arise organically and naturally, guided by our intuition when we sense anything the client may find difficult to discuss with us.

I might feel moved to say:

Th: Given the trauma you've experienced related to (e.g., race, gender, sexism, ageism), I wonder how it is to share with me? I encourage you to discuss anything that may cause you to feel I wouldn't understand you or make it difficult to share with me.

Ct: I'm glad you brought that up because I was wondering how I would discuss lesbian sex with you.

Th: How do you imagine I would react?

Ct: Well, you seem pretty straight, and you're older, so I imagine my sexual orientation would be very foreign to you.

Th: I'm so glad you're allowing us to talk about this. It's vital that you feel free and safe discussing anything that is important to you. I've worked with lesbian couples and helped them with their sexual issues. How is this for you to hear? It's also important that you feel you have a good fit with your therapist. Would you feel more comfortable with a lesbian therapist? (*Of course, if we do not feel we can be helpful, we need to be truthful.*)

Dispelling obstacles to closeness becomes paramount in therapy, and cultural disparities affect many clients. I spoke to Reiko Ikemoto-Joseph, LMFT, on this topic because of her expertise and personal experience regarding the significance of addressing cultural factors in therapy. She made some thought-provoking points: "Much has already been written about white privilege, but I think the best way to describe it is: 'never having occasion to consider one's own race.' For non-minority therapists who treat minority clients, this is a very important privilege to keep in mind. Treating this issue casually or as a non-issue definitely runs the risk of introducing shame into the therapeutic encounter." She recommended "encouraging therapists to continually examine their own biases, social privileges (including racial privileges) and be very mindful of the larger historical and societal forces at play for their clients. Sometimes we can focus myopically on attachment wounds or other intrapsychic conflicts at the expense of larger, real-world experiences that very often confer shame" (R. Joseph, personal communication, December 13, 2020).

If we are going to inquire into real world experiences involving painful memories, feelings, and associations with people who don't look like us or share our cultural background, we need to deal with any obstacles to such an exploration and welcome all feelings that surface. Many therapists find it challenging to invite complex feelings toward them, but we need to explore transference reactions and what we bring to the table with our clients. I want to re-emphasize how important it is that we resist self-devaluation as we encounter our client's anger toward us.

We hope to open doors, allowing us to enter into an "I-thou" instead of an "I-other" relationship. Reiko went on to say: "A subtle power dynamic often exists between a non-minority clinician and a minority client. Having been a minority my entire life, I can personally attest to the enormous shame attached to being perceived as 'the other' or 'the foreigner.' These associations will definitely surface in the therapeutic relationship, and a clinician would be wise and brave to address them early in the process." A power dynamic pervades the therapeutic process and each step we take toward collaboration, relinquishing the expert role, revealing out vulnerability and shortcomings, and learning from our clients helps to heal this power differential.

Reiko pointed out that I had used some language that could be perceived as a cultural stereotype in describing a client. She said, "Even though well-meaning and accurate, such language can be a source of shame." I changed that description. I regret any other instances like her example in the book, but my sensitivity to others is a work in progress, as I imagine it is for all of us.

Working with the pain of culture clashes

A young Hispanic mother with two small children found the courage in therapy to divorce her violently abusive husband. This decision came after a long, painful therapeutic process. As a result of the divorce, she lost her entire religious community. These people were her extended family for over a decade. Her closest friends, with whom she shared holidays and all special occasions, suddenly disappeared from her life (including attendants at her wedding and friends who witnessed her children's baptisms). Her story was heartbreaking to hear. These losses were overwhelming and tragic for her. It was tempting to judge her community, but splitting would deny her full reality, so we attended to her powerful complex feelings. We explored her horror, rage and intense love for those who had been her family for many years. Despite this terrible turn of events, her depression lifted, and she grew far healthier. But we couldn't deny the losses she suffered as a result. I felt awe at her courage.

A Chinese-American woman sat expectantly and quietly across from me. We soon spoke about the shame that made it hard for her to talk about herself.

Ct: I do not know what to say.

Th: Why don't you begin by telling me how you are suffering and what your hope for our work together.

Ct: I'm sad all the time.

Th: I feel for your deep sadness, and I'm glad you came here to get relief. I want that for you. I sense that you've had experiences that have made it difficult for you to focus on yourself. (*I spoke to her about the parasitic vine strangling a healthy tree, an outside force that was suffocating her.*) You cannot be happy until you are free to express yourself and feel safe, hopefully here with me.

She took a lot from that session, becoming aware of her shame and recognizing she was separate from it. She described feeling like a balloon with bright colors, lifting up and up, lighter and lighter. She smiled with tears of relief and said she felt hope for the first time in years. She and I developed a profound relationship. Over time, she told me how an ex-boyfriend and his friends raped her multiple times in a rural field. She'd never told anyone. Her whole family felt shame at her tragedy. Her culture expected her to nurse several male family members whom she despised in the final months of their lives, which took a grueling toll on her. She never complained. She told me she'd sometimes sit in the corner of her bathroom, trembling and contemplating suicide. The belief that she had no right to care about herself was the opposite of the freedom I was offering her.

Reiko commented, "These traumas unfolded within the larger context of rigid gender norms and societal expectations. The fact that you were **not** a part of her culture of origin was probably a huge relief and comfort to her. Sometimes being the "other" can be quite helpful clinically." This woman made significant changes in the dynamics of her marriage. We had some couples sessions, and I was delighted at the ways she began to assert herself. She also created a marvelous new business.

An Iranian-American woman highlighted some of the complexities and conflicts introduced by cultural differences:

Ct: Women have social roles in my culture, and you fulfill these expectations, or there is a big backlash. (*She listed several examples.*) I'm not able to express myself truthfully or bring my needs up for consideration.

Th: I'm very sad to hear this. I see that you pay a high price if you give voice to some of your wishes and feelings within your community. How is it to have a place here with me where no price will be paid for expressing yourself? I'm glad you're drawing closer to your boyfriend and wonder if you might find other safe relationships to be yourself while staying connected to family and old friends from your culture with whom you share so much history?

We need to refrain from assuming our values are superior or directing the decisions that belong to our clients. Reiko added: "The primacy of the self is an example of a Western bias embedded in many modalities. For many cultures, especially Asian cultures that are more collectivist in nature, this is not a given. Looking through this biased lens, we are more likely to interpret family loyalty (common especially among immigrant families) as 'enmeshment' or view Eastern values of filial piety as 'idealization.' In other words, we might inadvertently pathologize culturally sanctioned values."

The belief that our health depends on the freedom to recognize our feelings and express them in safe spaces undergirds the DEFT (Dynamic Emotion Focused Therapy) approach. But not all cultures value self-focusing or self-expression, and some religious beliefs conflict with the freedom to explore emotions. I make a point to separate self-caring from selfishness. Self-focusing to raise self-awareness increases responsiveness to others and decreases self-absorption, as in narcissism. Parallels exist between our work and Eastern meditative practice, noticing what arises in the moment from within the body and mind without judgment. If our work did not lead to greater expression of love, I would not do it.

How our clients navigate their choices remains very personal to each individual. Hopefully, people find creative ways to sustain their mental health as well as their sense of family, community, and tradition. But tragically, as with the young Hispanic-American mother, this is not always the case.

In Summary

No matter how exquisite our empathy, we can never enter the skin of another or replace what was lost. Even if we've had similar experiences, infinite variables shape how they impact us. The best we can offer is our desire to understand the unique individual before us, our humility in the face of what we do not know and need to learn, and our inexpressible caring for our fellow human beings. We offer a path out of suffering born of study, dedication, skill-building practice, a willingness to be vulnerable, learn from our clients, stretch ourselves, and use our best clinical intuition. Our cherished desire is to offer the highest quality relationship that the client can use as a model throughout one's life.

Our clients frequently long for twinship or a parent they never had. But hope lies in the discovery that the parent they long for lives inside them. Long-term healing rests in a commitment to self-care, involving an active engagement with one's feelings, needs, defenses and self-regulation. Our well-being also relies on a connection to community and consideration for others. An active engagement with oneself and others is not an idea or cognition but rather a day-to-day experience. Many of our clients have this new experience of safety and deep emotional connection for the first time in their lives with their therapist, who extends an invitation to a quality attachment relationship to enrich future relationships. Our clients hold that invitation in their hands. What will be their choice?

References

Bippus, A. M., & Young, S. L. (2005). Owning your emotions: Reactions to expressions of self-versus other-attributed positive and negative emotions. *Journal of Applied Communication Research*, *33*(1), 26–45. https://doi.org/10.1080/0090988042000318503

Bullard, D. (2015). Allan Schore on the science of the art of psychotherapy. *Psychotherapy.net News*. https://www.psychotherapy.net/interview/allan-schore-neuroscience-psychotherapy

Dyer, W. W. (2012). *The power of intention: Learning to co-create your world your way*. Hay House.

Frederickson, J. (2013). *Co-creating change: Effective dynamic therapy techniques*. Seven Leaves Press.

Gordon, T. (1975). *P.E.T., Parent effectiveness training: The tested new way to raise responsible children*. Plume.

Gottman, J., & Silver, N. (1999). *The seven principles for making marriage work*. Three Rivers Press.

Greenberg, L. S., & Paivio, S. C. (1997). *The practicing professional. Working with emotions in psychotherapy*. Guilford Press.

Main, T.F. (1957) The ailment. *British Journal of Medical Psychology* 30,129-145.

Main, T.F. (1989) *The ailment and other psychoanalytic essays*. Free Association Books.

Schore, A. (2012). *The Science of the Art of Psychotherapy*. W. W. Norton and Company.

Winnicott, D. W. (1948). Hate in the counter-transference. *The International Journal of Psychoanalysis*, 30, 69–74.

10

WHEN THE DAM BREAKS

Emotion focused therapists frequently feel pressure and responsibility to bring about emotional breakthroughs, sadly placing excessive burdens on themselves. Being motivated to grow is a good thing, but we don't want to strain to make something happen. When we fertilize the ground, seeds sprout without any pulling or pushing from us. It took me a long time to have faith in the principles I practice. Now I feel confident that if the client and I clear the obstacles on the path to the unconscious, and if it is the client's will to feel feelings, and if we focus on emotions when the barriers are low, the disowned parts of the self will step forward in amazing ways. Under the right conditions, we can trust the client's healing force to bring complex feelings to consciousness. The therapist's paradox is that we help to pave a path to emotional expression, but we have little to do with the parade that passes by, except to watch, listen, care, cheer, and offer guidance as needed. When the tapestry of the unconscious reveals itself, it is indeed a gift.

As feelings begin to surface, clients are surprised to discover aggressive impulses toward a beloved figure, which triggers intense guilt. They may retreat or shut down because that is how they learned to be loved. We want to help our clients stay open to their inner life and help them embrace the mixed feelings they had to hide. It's normal for therapists to

DOI: 10.4324/9780429399633-11

feel impatient with the process and become insistent and even demanding, like Little League parents pushing their kids to perform. We've all done that. Yet therapists don't make breakthroughs happen, and when we try, the process becomes forced, causing the unconscious to pull back again. Therapists can become discouraged, berating themselves because emotional unlockings elude them. We might believe our work is not good enough and feel ashamed.

Let's find encouragement in Leigh McCullough's research on affect processing, indicating that behavioral change can be observed at 25% emotional activation. Any moment when a client uncovers hidden, forbidden, or feared parts of oneself promotes change. These breakthroughs to intimacy are healing so long as there is emotional engagement. If someone shares something that's been repressed or suppressed, but the body is detached, the effect is far less than if the body is activated. Brene Brown's research (Brown, 2012) tells us that shared vulnerability leads to a greater connection to others. There is considerable research that connection to others leads to greater emotional and physical health (Smith & Weihs, 2019; Teo et al., 2013; Umberson & Montez, 2010). Therefore, every meaningful sharing of internal experience holds healing potential and deserves appreciation. We need to resist all-or-nothing thinking and celebrate the small unlockings as well as the large.

What Does it Mean to Feel a Feeling Fully?

Our clients expect minefields in the path of emotional expression. But once the client sees that the mines are from the past and have been disabled in the present, feelings feel safe to come forward. With encouragement, emotions will seek full expression. Opposing currents of complex feelings will pull us in different directions, but it helps us to sustain a focus on one feeling at a time.

Naming the Most Avoided Emotions

The most fertile path in psychotherapy often involves accessing the most difficult emotions. Someone who cries frequently may be defending against other feelings, and that person does not need encouragement to release more tears. The client needs our help with feelings they cannot access alone. We always want to ask, "Are you aware of other feelings besides this sadness as you talk about your husband?" Often, clients who have breakthroughs to rage will shut down because they have significant difficulty with grief and loss. Some possible interventions:

> *Th:* Could we see if there are other feelings besides your rage toward your dad? You mentioned some wonderful times with him and it was very hard for you to admit your anger. It will be so important to give attention to all that you feel.

Or:

> *Th:* What other feelings do you have besides this rage at your husband, who has now passed away? He never treated you like an equal, and yet you shared a rich history. Could we explore all your feelings toward him?

Awareness of Body Sensations that Accompany Feelings (See Figure 2.1)

We see in the examples below how these clients have developed a heightened awareness of body sensation:

> *Th:* What do you feel toward your wife as she runs errands for you so you'll have more time for your project? Do you notice any sensations in your body?
>
> *Ct:* Swelling in my chest *(expands his arms)*. It's love.

Another example:

> *Th:* Tell me how you feel as you tell me about your new ability to communicate with your family rather than avoid them?
>
> *Ct:* I guess you'd call it pride. I feel waves, pulses of warmth moving slowly.

A man described being humiliated by a coworker:

> *Ct:* I'm pissed off.
>
> *Th:* How does that feel in your body?
>
> *Ct:* Heat close to the belly that rises to my chest.

The ability to recognize the signals emanating from various organs and muscles is known as interoception, which impacts overall health. A deficit in interoception is linked to lower resilience, e.g., adaptation to stressors and trauma. Whether due to anxiety, ADHD, or organic factors, people who have difficulty focusing find it more challenging to track bodily sensations. I sometimes guide people through their bodies with attention to specific activation (e.g., noticing heart rhythms, breathing, body temperature, and activation in the muscles) to help them recognize sensations they would not otherwise notice. If I discover that someone has cognitive perceptual disruption or smooth muscle activation (see Anxiety, Chapter 7), I will do far more frequent body checks to avoid problematic symptoms of dysregulation. Some people become more anxious about focusing on the breath or disturbing sensations, and we may need to help them tolerate body awareness. One woman told me she could not follow her bodily sensations, and we discovered an organic explanation. If I had not accepted her stated limitation, she would have dropped out due to shame and appropriate anger.

Experiencing Impulses Attached to Emotions

We feel impulses as energy currents and muscle activation within the body that seek release through action. An absence of impulses is an absence of feelings. When impulses approach the surface, clients will typically feel muscle tension initially due to tightening around the impulse, a resistance to feelings. I usually suggest the client allow the impulses to move through the body and observe the flow of energy. As the impulses reach the extremities, we utilize fantasy to imagine how they want to release in actions. I might say to a client, "I'm not speaking to you, Carol, but rather to these energies in your body that are forces of nature. Can we ask these energies how they feel like moving and releasing from your body in a fantasy? Just keep noticing please."

Loving feelings may stir the desire to embrace; joy can make us feel like jumping; Sexual feelings can arouse an urge to kiss passionately, and fear can activate the impulse to run. Angry impulses move into the muscles of the outer extremities, such as an urge to raise our fists. "Portrayals" or visualizations of how the impulses would move out of the body add dimension and a deeper connection to the emotions. When a client shares the full experience of emotion with the therapist, anxiety and shame typically drop dramatically. Freedom to feel relaxes the body and is good for health. "The therapist's ability to affectively contain, mirror, or empathically resonate to rage, sadness and grief, and to undo the shame and/or guilt co-mingled with these emotions, may be the single most important curative factor in the therapy." (Neborsky, 2010).

One caveat

Please do not attempt a rage portrayal without training or supervision. We must be prepared to work with complex feelings when we portray rage. It is especially important that guilt over rage is identified and diminished. Clients can get frustrated when their feelings are stirred in therapy but remain unprocessed. Sometimes, this can't be avoided, but we can try to achieve as much closure as possible. It also takes a lot of practice to manage the time limitations in the therapy hour, as we don't want to start a deep uncovering with insufficient time.

Some therapists will not want to work with rage portrayals. I was one of them. I had to practice portrayals many times to understand their impact and feel confidence in the process. Even when my clients benefited significantly, it took quite awhile to trust in the value of the breakthrough process. Let's also remember that every therapeutic element we have discussed in this book has healing properties, according to my clients' feedback and the references I've cited. Therefore I caution therapists not to fixate on intense breakthroughs to the exclusion of all types of meaningful work. Many therapists tell me they have deepened their work with greater client satisfaction using the principles of this approach, although they have not incorporated rage portrayals significantly. Sometimes, they surprise themselves. One day, they begin to move toward fuller breakthroughs and do not turn back.

Therapist Discomfort with Emotions

Therapists often dread the emergence of long-repressed emotions. They wonder, "Will I be able to bear the feelings in my client or will intense emotions overwhelm me?" "What if my client loses control?" "What if emotion processing does irreparable damage?" "What if my inadequacies become obvious?" When we fear unfamiliar emotional terrain, we may shift into the comfort of diversification, wordiness, and headiness. Let's say a man recalls the sound of his alcoholic father closing the door to the garage after a night at the bar. The client may be close to a breakthrough, but the therapist who becomes uneasy, asks, "What do you *think* that meant to you (intellectualizing, generalizing)? There were many elements at work, given the upheaval after your family lost their home (rationalizing)?" We want to avoid left-brain words like "think" or "assess" to encourage feelings. Due to anxiety, the therapist can unconsciously shift away from raw feelings. This chapter aims to provide a compass as you head out to sea.

Our instincts to pace ourselves as we work with intense feelings can be useful when we need more skill development, support, or inner work to increase our tolerance for emotional expression. I remember falling off a surfboard and slamming my face onto the ocean floor, never realizing sand could feel like brick. I've had similar sensations when I tried processing trauma-laden emotions without sufficient preparation. Once I'd been so pleased that I could help a woman feel rage for the first time, but she never came back! I felt devastated. I understood what happened after a follow-up phone call. Time ran out before I could adequately address her guilt over her rage. When clients confront their fury directly for the first time and believe this feeling turns them into a monster, they may leave the session with worsened symptoms and self-hatred.

Some comments I might have said to the client I lost:

"You yearned to be close to your mother, but it was never possible. You're lashing out at her because of your enormous loss, and your rage wants to stop your pain. I'm glad you could release your rage, but I know it very difficult for you to look at these feelings. It's so vitally important that you allow yourself to keep looking at your feelings for having destroyed your mother." *She loves her mother and needs to access her love to feel at peace with herself.*

"Might we have compassion for your pain and accept your natural reaction without judgment or guilt?"

"Your guilt tells us how deeply you care for your mother while hating her for the gashing emotional wound she inflicted on you. Despite your pain in this relationship, you find it within yourself to continue to love her. Could we take a look at how you would express your love toward your mother, having unleashed your fury on her body?"

Why should we encourage people to release their impulses toward the figure who hurt them? This therapy faces truth and reality to the greatest degree possible so there is no place within ourselves we have to hide. Sometimes people say they want to hit a coffee table. But we know the impulse is toward a specific person rather than an inanimate object. These feelings can be faced within a compassionate relationship. For some extremely fragile clients, we may start with the impulses toward the table and build the capacity to face feelings toward the person.

Love is the flip side of rage. People who matter the most have the greatest power to hurt us. When people connect to the love beneath their rage, they soften toward themselves and the person who hurt them. Linking their rage to thwarted love brings forth a sense of poignancy and loss, and makes rage more acceptable. If I could impart one message to my colleagues, it would be: rage and love always co-exist with trauma histories. One feeling does not cancel out the other, though clients often fear that complex feelings cannot co-exist. Rage work will fail if our clients deny their complex feelings.

The therapist needs to leave time to focus on defenses against guilt over rage. We do not want this guilt to turn into self-hatred or self-punishment. Guilt and love are intertwined, and reaching the love that exists on the other side of rage provides the most profound healing. If a client feels rage and then shuts down, we need to do our most active defense work. I let my clients know that their recovery depends on access to all their feelings, which inevitably leads to more profound love.

What are My Most Avoided Feelings as a Therapist?

Dan Siegel has said, "Narrative integration is more than just making up a story—it is a deep, bodily and emotional process of sorting through the muck in which we've been stuck" (Siegel, 2007, pp. 308–309). Depth emotion work is intersubjective. Either partner may confront one of their "stuck in the muck" moments and feel scared, ashamed, profoundly sad, sexually aroused, or enraged. As I look back on my journey, there can never be enough preparation to eliminate all risk and fear.

My toughest challenges have been absorbing very positive or sexual feelings toward me, and processing rage. I kept pulling away from my discomfort, which makes me sad, because I left the client behind, even unintentionally. On the other hand, sometimes I felt proud for tolerating my fear and sticking with uncomfortable emotions. Once a man expressed feeling attracted to me, and my chest tightened. I could have veered and said, "Yes, you were telling me about the time you started dating Haley." Instead, I asked if he felt aroused? He said he was. I asked myself, "Why shouldn't I stay with these sensations when I stay with all other sensations related to feelings?" So I pressed on and asked about the sensations that accompanied his aroused state? He began to go into graphic detail, and at one point, I had the uneasy sense that our dialogue was gratifying him, and defenses were operating. During a breakthrough, feelings move through the body, and new feelings emerge. But my client seemed stuck in a groove, so I asked, "Are you aware of other feelings? I sense that your sexual feelings are overwhelming other feelings that are important for you to access." He had a history of seeing prostitutes and acting out sexually. He began noticing that rage was also rising. He didn't understand it. I encouraged him to follow that feeling too, and as anger intensified in his body, I encouraged him to release those impulses in a fantasy. He then felt the desire to rape me violently, and soon I transformed into his mother, who had been emotionally absent throughout his childhood. He was forcing her into the union he craved. I was glad that I'd stuck with those difficult sensations earlier in the session, as he would not have accessed the material that allowed him to link his compulsive sexual behavior to his futile efforts to gain his mother's love. Grief broke through. This session had a profound impact on his relationships with women.

Here's an example of a breakthrough of intensely positive feelings, in which I had to resist my urges to take the spotlight off myself and damp down too much praise. My elderly client had made surprising changes. She'd become more attuned to others, became willing to show vulnerability in her relationships, and she risked traveling to places that would have been too frightening for her before.

Th: Wow, Beatrice, it's awesome that you took that trip by yourself! Isn't that exciting?

Ct: Yes! I feel like a kid who just won a prize in a spelling bee or something. I used to gulp down my food, and it was like chewing a steak and enjoying every mouthful.

Th: Relishing every bite.

Ct: Yes! Awake and alive. And letting my sense of humor come out with my friends too.

Th: Let's take a look and see if anything feels new here, in this moment.

Ct: Well, certainly the comfort, the peace. I am peaceful about being 84 (*she used to have an intense fear of dying*), about being here and saying, "You're here. Let's not screw it up. Let's just go with it. See where we go. See what happens. Let's have some adventures. Let's see what's out there." As wonderful as I feel, you have to feel fabulous.

Th: I do. (*I notice some resistance to shifting the focus to me.*)

Ct: You have to feel even more fabulous than I because—

Th: I don't know about that. (*Cutting her off, deflecting, and she pushes back.*)

Ct: Well, but Susan, please hear this. Alone, I never could have done it. So you took me from there, and you brought me to here. I thank you from the deepest corner of my heart. I've had therapy throughout the years, and I have accomplished more with you, Susan. You don't permit crap from me, which was different from the other therapists, but you really—

Th: (*Again, I took the focus off of me, intellectualized and deflected her compliment.*) Well, I interrupted any part of you that could hurt you.

Here, I might have asked her how she felt sharing such positive feelings toward me, being so free to express her appreciation, warmth, and caring? I might have allowed myself to absorb her appreciation. I had worked hard to help her. Why not linger with that lovely, happy feeling? This woman started with strong distancing defenses and typically did not acknowledge other people. I might have stayed with her feelings and mine as we celebrated our relationship. But I didn't. She persisted.

Ct: Yeah. Yeah. Because you don't let me. When I'm here, and I don't want to be here, and I move away, that's when you say, "Let's stay here." And we stay there. And you bring me right back so that I can look at myself and see that I'm not horrible. I'm basically adorable. I've found love. (*We both giggle. She was adorable when she said she was adorable.*)

Th: So that you and I can have a true relationship with the true you, and embrace who you are, and not reject any part of you. That's what I would interrupt, any part of you that would reject or deny us this experience.

Ct: Maybe two or three visits back, I thought, "I really could say goodbye to you." And as we spent the session, I really couldn't. Now, I know that I can say goodbye. No, not goodbye. Au revoir. That's lovely. Because something will come up. Maybe it won't. But if it does, I know I have my friend, my dearest friend to whom I can come. We'll walk through it together again. And I'll be right back here. But again, you have, I don't know if you know just how good you are. (*Again, she wanted me to absorb her gift of caring and gratitude.*) But I'm here to tell you, Susan, you are good.

Th: You touch me, Beatrice.

Ct: You are very good, my dearest friend.

Th: That is so dear of you to say that.

Ct: But you and I know it's true. And if I was saying it to you and you didn't believe me— (*how interesting that she picked up my difficulty acknowledging her appreciation*).

Th: Well, I only know it through this kind of exchange, Beatrice. And you allow me to feel it, and I so appreciate that. (*I make an effort to absorb her compliment and feel it.*)

Ct: Well, I want you to feel it because I want you to know if you can do this for me, you're going to do it for the next one. And the one who was here before. (*She was giving me the acknowledgment that I would typically be offering to my clients. I felt like we had switched seats, as it should be at times.*)

Th: Isn't that amazing, this change, this circle?

Ct: It's this circle we talk about that runs around between us. It's like we're on a track, and we come to you, and then we come back to me, and we're circling around. (*She moves her hands between us in a circling motion, suggesting the intersubjectivity of our relationship.*)

Th: That's exactly right.

Ct: It's the connection that's there. So that circle really can't be broken. (*Next, she talks about going out of her way to be responsive to a friend. Her self-absorption would have prevented this kind of empathy before.*) Today, my joy at telling Patricia to call Betsy because I knew Betsy was hurting is very special. It's getting outside of me and not just being me but being part of my community of friends. (*Importantly, she describes how she resolved her relationship with her son, from whom she'd been distant. She had been very critical in the past that he wasn't more attentive to her.*)

Ct: I've come to terms with him. I love him. And he loves me. He loves me, dearly. There is no question. I know if the chips are down, and I really need him, I call him, and he will be there. I'm growing up. (*I felt very fulfilled at this moment. She had risen above her projections onto her son that he didn't care about her. She saw beyond her splitting and saw him as a flawed human who loved her.*)

Th: Knowing that you are loved and lovable and that you can live with human limitations and, therefore, you have so much more to give.

Ct: The more you give, the more you get. There's a part of me that thinks, "Are you sure you want to leave her?" But I know I have to grow up and go.

Shifting Gears

As I study hundreds of psychotherapy sessions, I sometimes see missed opportunities to take the next step toward feelings. The therapist has succeeded in working with the barrier in the forefront (e.g., lowering anxiety, shame, or a defense) but does not shift gears and focus on feelings. Keeping in mind that "timing is everything," these opportune moments may pass quickly. The therapist may be avoidant or believes the barriers are higher than they are in actuality. Perhaps anxiety reduction work absorbed an entire session, but the therapist reached satisfactory anxiety regulation within fifteen minutes.

Good timing of interventions

The checklist below will guide the therapist in determining good timing and client readiness to begin focusing on feelings. How do we know if the alliance is favorable to increase exposure to feelings? When is self-compassion strong enough to activate the will to face feelings? Do we sense when the will comes online? A client may say, "I'm ready" or "I want to do this," but the therapist may lag behind. We can stall the process and even stop it entirely if we become distracted or retreat during this phase. When we turn to the left-brain, we'll slow the unearthing of emotions (e.g., using phrases like "What do you think?" or "How would you explain...?") We want to use right-brain words in this phase, like, "What feelings do you sense?" or "Stay with your body as you immerse yourself in this experience." "How do you imagine these energies want to be released?" or, "Are you aware of images?" Once we begin focusing on feelings, we may experience a rapid unlocking, or a barrier slows it down. We may need a few moments or longer (depending on the strength of the resistance, anxiety, shame or guilt). before we reestablish the capacity to bear feelings.

First Breakthrough: Sadness for the Cost of Defenses

When is self-compassion strong enough to activate the will to face feelings? As clients recognize the internal operations that have silenced their feelings, they realize the extent of their deprivation over a lifetime of disconnection from their emotions. Typically, tears of regret and pain follow. This breakthrough to sadness is compassion for oneself and often mobilizes the will to be free to feel. If the client's awareness of the defenses are cognitive only and the body appears detached, the will to risk feelings will probably remain dormant.

Checklist for Breakthrough Work

1 Proceed only with permission to focus on feelings
2 Remain vigilant to an uptick in defenses
3 Be on the alert to anxiety outside a low-moderate range
4 Explore impulses slowly
5 Emphasize the exploration of complex feelings
6 The Burial Fantasy
7 Treat the numbing of grief and love after rage as a defense
8 Make meaning of the breakthrough process collaboratively

Proceed Only with Permission to Focus on Feelings

If the client agrees to feeling-focused work but blocks your efforts at every turn, you do not have implicit permission. We can check it out:

> *Th:* I get the sense that a part of you wants to connect with your feelings toward your dad, but another part changes the subject each time we move closer. Could we ask that part of you that changed course to speak to us and tell us how it feels about what we're doing here? (*This invitation will help reveal the resistance so we can work with it consciously.*)

Permission to explore feelings is active when a client brings up an emotionally laden experience and shares bodily sensations. Sustain the focus on feelings toward one person. Bring the experience to life by inquiring about details of time, place, textures, smells and sounds. Examples of trauma-laden memories recalled by my clients: the red plaid shirt her grandfather was wearing when he fondled her as he lay on his bed; the smell of the pine floor as her brother played with her; the sound of the garage door closing when dad came home from the bar. Recapturing these memory fragments awakens the senses and stirs dormant feelings. The more we can revisit the past, the more we can leave it behind.

Remain Vigilant to an Uptick in Defenses

Resistance has a voice and a velocity. Mild, tactical defenses, like diversification or some nervous laughter, may not require our attention. However, others need our full focus like, "You're making a big deal out of nothing," or "I don't see the point in what we're doing." Dismiss the more significant obstacles at your peril because they can morph into misattunements. Following are examples of dealing with a variety of defenses:

Generalizing, Rationalizing, Displacement, Denial, and Splitting

> *Th:* How do you feel toward your Dad?
>
> *Ct:* I feel angry. I see him with a stick hitting me. He was always nice and smiling, never angry, so his whippings came out of nowhere.

Th: You expected kindness, but he betrayed your trust.

Ct: And I feel terrible (*vague*). I guess parents aren't perfect (*generalizing, rationalizing*).

Th: You said you feel angry when you think about this now (*returning to the most avoided feeling*).

Ct: I feel angry at my mother, not my father, even though he was the one that did this (*displacement of anger toward father onto mother*).

Th: But your mother didn't put a gun to his head. He picked up the stick (*undoing the displacement*).

Ct: I know. But my dad worked hard, and she would start telling him all kinds of things, and he would lose it (*rationalizing dad's actions*).

Th: Might we stay with this instance in which he becomes violent and loses control? You're just a little girl, and your father, who you looked up to and relied upon, is suddenly turning into a monster, losing it and attacking you. When you just stay with that reality, how do you feel? (*Returning to her avoided feelings*).

Ct: Scared. I was frightened.

Th: You must have been terrified!

Ct: I was frightened, but I don't remember being angry.

Th: How about right now? (*Bringing her back to the present. Take note when people say what they don't feel. When the client brings up a feeling and negates it, the feeling still comes to mind. Often, when we say we don't feel something, we do.*) *The session continues:*

Be on the Alert to Anxiety Outside a Low To Moderate Range

Th: You don't remember being angry but how about right now, in this moment?

Ct: I am angry. I would be angry at anyone who touches a child, even a slap.

Th: And this was far more than a slap. How much anger do you feel toward your dad for striking you? (*Helping to identify the intensity of the anger*).

Ct: A lot!

Th: So how do you feel that anger in your body, in total honesty, because this is what will help you feel less anxious *(linking her goals to emotional expression)*.

Ct: I feel it in my legs.

Th: What do you notice in your legs?

Ct: They feel weak, rubbery. I was probably scared stiff. I want to run, but I can't (*Jelly legs indicates smooth muscle activation and significant anxiety.*)

Th: You froze in fear. Any child would freeze. It's horrifying to be terrorized when you're small and defenseless. And right now, would you say you are freezing up as if your dad was here, as though you are still seven or eight? You're freezing up with me. (*Client nods in agreement. We work on her anxiety until it lowers, and then we proceed.*) What if you let yourself feel the energy in your legs. What about feeling it without becoming paralyzed? (*Providing alternatives to anxiety.*)

Ct: I would have kicked him. Or tried to defend myself, punched him.

Th: Is that what your legs feel like doing?

Ct: Yeah, kicking him in his legs and taking the stick from his hand and shoving him (*breakthrough of impulse as she begins to attack him violently in retaliation*).

Explore Impulses Slowly

Fully attending to a feeling gives it value. Explore impulses a step at a time, like watching a film with all its imagery. Rushing conveys we want to avoid rather than embrace feelings, although we have to be mindful of the time left in a session. Always check to see where the activation occurs in the body. When clients tell a story with no bodily activation, they are in defense. When this occurs, we might say:

Th: You can name your feeling, but sadly you don't have the freedom to feel your impulses. If we leave your feelings and impulses locked up inside you, they do damage to your body and spirit. You have tightness in your chest. Your chest isn't happy, and tension is unhealthy. Your stress can affect your digestion. Would you be willing to invite those energies in your chest to move through and out of your body for the sake of your health and well being?

Ct: I'm willing to try.

Th: Great. Where are the impulses in your body now?

Ct: They're in my upper arms and chest.

Th: Good. I'm not speaking to you right now, Jack. I'm speaking to your impulses. If they had no restraints and could do no wrong, how do they feel like releasing from your body?

Ct: I want to pound (*beginning of release of impulses*).

Th: Who are you pounding? Where are you pounding? With what velocity?

Tightness in the jaw may release as a biting impulse. In one client, muscle tension that created a tight band around the head (she was prone to migraines) released as an impulse to bash her mother's head. A choking sensation may release as an impulse to choke. When we give our full attention to a feeling, we give it value.

Ct: I'm pounding my brother. He's on the ground. I'm punching him.

Th: Where are you punching him?

Ct: Mostly in his stomach and chest. I'm screaming and kicking.

Th: Well, that scream is your desire to lash out, your fury. What if that fury toward him released out of your body fully?

Ct: I'd punch him for 15 minutes, just pounding, I'd bang his head on the floor, getting it all out. (*We give the client the time needed to release the impulses completely. He pounds and kicks hard for several minutes.*)

Th: And what's the end? What would you want to do to release every ounce of it? In all honesty, every last bit of it?

Ct: I would hit his head on the floor until he lost consciousness.

Th: What's happening to his head?

Ct: It makes a noise. Cracking his skull. I don't feel like killing him, though.

Sometimes clients don't want a quick death because they want to torture the person as they felt tortured over the years. Or, they may be defending against or denying their murderous impulses. In one case, the client couldn't bear to separate from her father. We pursue the exploration to gain more clarity.

Th: Cracking his skull on the floor. And what has happened to make that noise? You are slamming his head against the hardwood floor, and you hear this cracking sound. What has happened to him? (*Facing the true intent of the animal impulse.*)

Ct: His skull is open. There's a crack in the back of it. He's almost dead then. I see him out of breath, almost dead, no life. And then I take his head and do this again (*slamming motion*), and it cracks open. Now he's dead.

Emphasize the Exploration of Complex Feelings

We want to encourage the expression of all feelings. Feelings flow like currents of a river. After a rage breakthrough, defenses often block other feelings, but the work becomes problematic if the complex feelings of guilt, love, and grief are left unprocessed. I might say, "You've come so far in your work. It's vitally important that we stay open to all your feelings, or you won't have the relief you seek. We know that rage is not all that you feel toward your dad." (For research on the value of processing complex emotions, see Abbass & Town, 2013; Abbass et al., 2017; Johansson et al., 2014.) The burial fantasy is one powerful means to bring about the integration of painful, conflicted feelings.

The Burial Fantasy

I typically will ask, "How do you envision laying the body to rest?" When we uncover murderous impulses in therapy, the client may shut down the emerging grief attached to the rage, guilt over rage, love, and loss of a beloved parent. Visualizing a burial fantasy can be a powerful tool to help the client connect with their love and loss, leading to a greater sense of resolution and the ability to leave the past behind. There may be a series of "final goodbyes" needed before a person can move forward. Each time I write or speak about this phase of this work, I know how foreign and even distasteful it will be for therapists who have little exposure to the power of this process. Therapists may be surprised how many of their current clients might uncover similar impulses and fantasies with guidance and find great relief and healing from expressing these unconscious feelings. In the following example, we see the power of the burial fantasy and the profound resolution of trauma that resulted.

A physically abusive mother slammed her son across the face with her open palms, full force. She covered him in shame, and he expected all women to obliterate him. He had left his wife, and we were working on rage toward his girlfriend. He had symptoms of severe anxiety, detachment and distancing when he began therapy. He had progressed considerably:

Th: So, do you have a sense of what that anger feels like toward her?

Ct: It just feels like a whole-body experience of energy throughout my body, in my arms, in my head, everywhere that wants to snuff her out.

Th: How does the energy feel like doing that (*encouraging connection to his impulses*)?

Ct: I'm getting big. Just grabbing hold of her shoulders and pushing her through the earth, and like driving her into the earth. And I'm just pushing her whole body through the earth, and I'm just pushing it down and driving it down like a corkscrew. And I'm just like trying to hold it there. And my hands are all gnarled like this—like taking a big, giant hammer and smashing the bricks, like that. She's underneath and just smashing, and smashing, and smashing the bricks. Crumbling the bricks that she's underneath. Umm.

Th: She's underneath bricks?

Ct: Yes, and I'm smashing and smashing, and like there's dust coming up, and I'm just holding her down under there, like basically sealing it and sealing the hole that she's in. Until I finally hit one brick that is in touch with her body, and it's just like (*makes exploding sound*) it obliterates, it obliterates the whole thing.

Th: Her. It obliterates her (*making it personal*).

Ct: Yeah, it obliterates her.

Making a Transfer to Other Figures

I ask, "And is there more?" Even though he had destroyed his girlfriend, he became aware of new waves of rage. I asked if other people came to mind. He had associations with his wife *and his mother. He envisioned ripping them apart, chopping them to pieces with a machete, and then swirling the pieces of all three women into a tornado until it exploded. He became afraid of his rage impulses. Although he had never attacked anyone physically and rarely lost control, he once threw an object and broke it. We discover he fears becoming violent like his mother. I remind him that he does not have an impulse problem like his mother.*

Th: You're afraid you can't hold your rage with me as your mother could not hold her rage with you? Yet you are no longer a child alone, at the mercy of your mother. Your trauma has passed. You have far more awareness and resources than your mother. You are not her.

Ct: (*Sighing respiration as feelings rise to the surface*). Some part of me feels like that, like it's just bringing up so much anger that I just umm—(*He suggests feeling overwhelmed by the intensity of his rage, and I remind him of our relationship to help soothe and regulate his fears.*)

Th: May I suggest you make eye contact with me, Brett, just try looking into my eyes, to know that I'm here with you? I know this fury is gigantic toward these three women because you feel attacked. (*Normalizing his fury by pointing to the mix of hurt, pain, and love that ignited such fierce protest. His anxiety relates to shame and guilt over his retaliatory rage, which he fears he cannot control.*)

Th: Would you want to express to your mother's departing spirit why your rage was inevitable (*helping him to accept his rage*)?

Ct: I wanted to annihilate you, Mom, because of the way you treated me... your complete lack of respect, your cruelty.

Th: You annihilated her as she annihilated you. How would you envision laying to rest the bodies of your mother, your girlfriend, and your wife? (*His following comments express the serenity he feels after releasing his storm of feelings and clearing the debris of his trauma. He finds a new wholeness as he picks up the pieces he values about these relationships.*)

Ct: I envision going somewhere by myself and one by one just digging a hole, a proper hole on a green hill, trees.

Th: A peaceful, serene place.

Ct: (*He speaks slowly, tenderly.*) Yes, the ocean is in the background. I dust off their clothes, smooth their hair, kissing them, lovingly covering them in brightly colored flower petals, dirt, and tightly packed stones to seal their graves.

Th: Would you be willing to just stay with what you feel there?

Ct: It feels somber but resolved—some kind of resolution. The thing that's coming to mind is, "I just don't need you to make me feel whole anymore. But if I go deeper, it's, "Thank you. Thank you for helping me." (*He fights back his tears. His cheeks look puffy.*) I'm sad for myself that this numbing mechanism takes hold of me in this way. (*Preventing a release of his sobs.*)

Th: Yes. Me too. Do we honor your feelings coming up at this moment? You want to cry.

Ct: I notice some heaviness and pressure in my chest. (*He begins to reflect on his newfound ability to notice the numbing mechanism that automatically shuts down his feelings, a type of breakthrough unto itself.*) *Because* I'm just sitting here bearing witness to the thing. I'm not even controlling the thing. It's just doing it. If I'm honest, I feel some happiness coming up, like, "Okay, this mechanism is losing some grip." Just a lot of sensation in my chest. And like, wow, battle-weary from all the struggle to be me.

Th: Um, hmm.

Ct: It feels tender, like softness. And some real sensitivity toward myself and these efforts to just allow me to be what I am. (*He sheds tears of compassion for himself.*)

Th: Right, just to be you, just to be all of you, with this crazy thing that attacks you, just to allow yourself to be where you are, noticing, taking pleasure in noticing all of this. I can see where that brings up sadness for you because you haven't had a lot of that space just to be safely you. Just to be safely yourself.

Ct: This is the first time I can remember feeling the mechanism itself as painful. The mechanism itself is now standing out. It's standing out. (*Brett is now becoming fully aware of the pain and loss caused by his distancing, detaching, numbing defenses.*) I'm starting to see it as highlighted, as painful, more painful than feeling all the other things that are underneath it. I need this anger. I need this force of anger to protect this work I'm doing. (*He makes a significant point. The pain caused by his defenses is far greater than the emotional pain they attempt to cover.*)

Th: Right. You need all of your feelings, Brett. You need the sadness too. You need all of your feelings. But right now, you're just getting super aware of all of those forces that would stop you from connecting and being at peace with what's inside you.

Ct: Yeah, it's just like taking off a mask, the emergence of something long overdue. I can feel sort of sad and happy at the same time for myself.

Treat the Numbing of Grief and Love after Rage as a Defense

In Brett's case, he immediately recognized his numbing mechanism as a defense, so I didn't have to point it out. His observing capacity remained active, and he stayed engaged with himself. If he had shut down and aligned with his numbing mechanism, I would have actively raised awareness of the defense and begun to activate compassion and will to move past this blockage. The unconflicted love that Brett began to experience toward the significant women in his life began to undo his guilt and fear over his rage impulses.

Guilt over rage impulses

If Brett had protested when his mother smacked him in the face as a child, she would have beaten him harder. He needed to repress rage and numb out to survive. Yet, urges to retaliate when attacked are innately human. Those who strive to be "good" and "obedient" judge their animalistic impulses and feel guilt for these feelings. Repeated exposures to complex feelings are often profoundly curative in resolving trauma. However, some cases will remain long-term, and we should not have inflated expectations about all cases. In most cases, this type of processing leads to symptom reduction and much improved relationships. The client becomes clear that the wounded child had to feel intense retaliatory rage, and the guilt reveals the presence of love. No crime exists. We were seeking union all along.

When a woman who had loved a series of male abusers finally told me forcefully that she felt angry at her current partner, her next thoughts were, "I feel guilty. He's been through so much. He couldn't help himself." She asked me, "So what good will it do to feel my anger?" I said, "Without your anger, you've lost a limb, and you're asking me to help you to walk upright. Without your anger, you will have no protection."

A variety of factors ease unwarranted guilt over rage

1 Internalizing the therapist's empathy for the rage
2 Normalizing the rage—"Who wouldn't feel rage under these circumstances?
3 Reframing the client's view of rage
It's a stunning new perspective for many clients to realize that rage only destroys when it leads to acting out or discharge. They can safely notice rage impulses within the body, a harmless energy. If more parents could work internally with their rage, anxiety and shame, far fewer kids would witness violence in their homes. Rage is an inevitable, hard-wired protest against separation and loss, a conquering force against threats to attachment and closeness. A protector and fighter for justice, rage mobilizes the self in vital and necessary ways.
4 Welcoming and encouraging the grief that follows rage
5 Discovering the intense love that lay beneath the rage

Avoiding the pain of facing the losses that we cannot recover

Some people will access murderous impulses but want to torture a caregiver endlessly, with no conclusion or resolution. One female client had enormous rage breakthroughs to her alcoholic father, but she resisted the burial. I asked her to help me understand. She didn't want to say goodbye and give up hope for their relationship. Once we brought her avoidance to consciousness, she painfully allowed herself to bury him. Her desire to keep her father alive stoked a fantasy that he would finally produce the love she craved. But this would not be reality. She found it agonizing to confront the fact that "Dad and I missed so many golden opportunities to be close, and they can never be realized in this lifetime." When defenses operate against facing this loss, we draw awareness to the defense and its cost.

New emotional freedoms highlight the losses of the past

As clients discover they no longer need to internalize, repress, or convert their rage to anxiety and shame, they experience the liberation that is possible. These realizations also highlight what could have been possible had their early relationships been different or had they been more aware of themselves earlier in their lives. These discoveries often bring up waves of new pain.

Make Meaning of the Breakthrough Process Collaboratively

This phase ushers in a right/left brain integration. The feeling parts of the mind meet the reflective and cognitive parts of the mind. This review is a time for memory reconsolidation and making meaning together as therapeutic partners. Repressed memories may have arisen, which may change the client's perspectives of past events. I mentioned the client who remembered his abusive father had carved a special toy for him. He recognized his loving feelings toward his dad for the first time in many years. Parents can be seen as complex human beings, just as clients come to see themselves as multi-dimensional, no longer needing to be viewed as all good or bad but rather as flawed and valuable humans.

Sometimes therapists do a lot of interpreting in this phase, but I prefer to actively listen to the meaning the client makes of the experience. "There is accumulating evidence that both the in-session activation of specific, relevant emotions and the cognitive exploration and elaboration of the significance and meaning of these emotions are important for therapeutic change" (Whelton, 2004, p. 58). It's helpful to reflect together on the barriers to feelings that presented themselves pre-breakthrough, the insights gained from the breakthrough, and how the client would want to use these insights in their current lives. What might emerge? Maybe someone decides they want to express some feelings to a family member, and we may discuss how to go about this to get the best results. There are a multitude of possibilities for change that may rise to consciousness.

We embrace our clients in totality when we accompany them through the full range of their emotions, providing an experience of unconditional acceptance. The therapeutic relationship generates self-love, which fertilizes the capacity to love others. Once complex feelings can be freely processed, only love remains.

References

Abbass, A. A., & Town, J. M. (2013). Key clinical processes in intensive short-term dynamic psychotherapy. *Psychotherapy, 50*(3), 433–437. https://doi.org/10.1037/a0032166

Abbass, A., Town, J., Ogrodniczuk, J., Joffres, M., & Lilliengren, P. (2017). Intensive short term dynamic psychotherapy trial therapy: Effectiveness and role of "unlocking the unconscious". *Journal of Nervous and Mental Disease, 205*(6), 453–457. https://doi.org/10.1097/NMD.0000000000000684

Brown, B. (2012). *Daring greatly: How the courage to be vulnerable transforms the way we live, love, parent, and lead.* Penguin.

Johansson, R., Town, J., & Abbass, A. (2014). Davanloo's intensive short-term dynamic psychotherapy in a tertiary psychotherapy service: Overall effectiveness and association between unlocking the unconscious and outcome. *PeerJ*. 2. 10.7717/peerj.548.

Neborsky, Robert J. (2010). *The collected writings of Robert J. Neborsky, MD.* Unlocking Press.

Siegel, D. J. (2007). *The mindful brain: Reflection and attunement in the cultivation of well-being (Norton series on interpersonal neurobiology).* Norton.

Smith, T., & Weihs, K. (2019). Emotion, social relationships, and physical health: Concepts, methods, and evidence for an integrative perspective. *Psychosomatic Medicine, 81*(8), 681–693. https://doi.org/10.1177/0022146510383501

Teo, A. R., Choi, H., & Valenstein, M. (2013). Social relationships and depression: Ten-year follow-up from a nationally representative study. *PloS ONE, 8*(4), Article e62396. https://doi.org/10.1371/journal.pone.0062396

Umberson, D., & Montez, J. K. (2010). Social relationships and health: A flashpoint for health policy. *Journal of Health and Social Behavior, 51*, S54–S66. https://doi.org/10.1177/0022146510383501

Whelton, W. J. (2004). Emotional processes in psychotherapy: Evidence across therapeutic modalities. *Clinical Psychology & Psychotherapy, 11*(1), 58–71. https://doi.org/10.1002/cpp.392

11

THE PEOPLE WHISPERER

What are the qualities of a people whisperer? This novel question entered my mind after watching a mesmerizing film about a famous horse whisperer, a trainer whose intuitive communication style transforms wild horses into cooperative companions in a relatively short time. He does not "break" these animals but works his magic by creating safety and respect. One of the most famous practitioners, Monty Roberts, travels worldwide to teach his skills to professionals working with victims, violent offenders, autistic children, and substance abusers. I envision "people whisperers" as healers who tap into an instinctive, inspired, and intuitive interpersonal realm. Skills, techniques, methods, and protocols provide therapists with an orientation, but we need relational capacities that transcend any skill set. I shudder when I think of those times I have used evidence-based protocol that backfired without the guidance of my intuition.

"A tug-of-war exists regarding the validity of clinical intuition compared with evidence-based approaches" (Marks-Tarlow, 2012, p. 37). A quote attributed to Einstein may help to resolve this conflict: "The intuitive mind is a sacred gift and the rational mind is a faithful

DOI: 10.4324/9780429399633-12

servant. We have created a society that honors the servant and has forgotten the gift." We must prioritize the therapist's clinical intuition, existing outside of our direct control and arising mostly from the unconscious. When a client shifted his eyes for a millisecond, I felt concerned and lurched forward in my seat and asked if he was all right. He said he'd had a fainting sensation similar to other times he had fainted and gone to the emergency room. We know the speed of light, but what is the speed of intuition? My client's anxiety had escalated rapidly in response to closeness and it fell back to normal almost as quickly with some soothing words, reflection and a bit of humor. Who knows what would have happened if it had been ignored? Much of the intuitive, lightning-fast responses that occur between mother and infant take place in our offices too, as we sense the infant within the adult client. When humans feel secure, they will push boundaries and seek the new, as when my client said at a family gathering, "Let's put this family dynamic BS aside for a second and act like we're just all adults." This kind of directness was unprecedented in a family who spoke banalities to each other. A stunning shift occurred between them, and they enjoyed each other. The human relationship is a living entity that needs spontaneity, flexibility, humor, creativity, and imagination to express its uniqueness, vitality, and potential to grow.

Buck Brannaman, a third-generation horse whisperer, teaches that mammals have instinctive forces that allow them to trust, relate, and become their best selves, depending on how people relate to them. Buck is a rare breed. He's an open, vulnerable, wise cowboy who transcended horrific trauma at the fists of his violent father. His devoted foster parents rescued him, and Buck became determined that he would not inflict the agony of his childhood upon other living beings. He used his early pain to approach wild and unruly horses from a place of consummate compassion, using gentle, kind, and confident non-verbal cues. I watched Buck mount a formerly fierce and frenzied horse. My jaw dropped when the pair glided at a sideways angle across a majestic Montana mountainous terrain at sunset, as though they were born to be together. Another untamed horse with no halter abruptly fell behind Buck, matching his pace exactly. When Buck paused, the horse paused in perfect synchronicity. When I walk with my husband

and his pace slows, I think of the horse that is eager to move ahead but slows down to be a partner.

You Have to Give and Take

I had an encounter with a newly tamed horse while visiting an old friend. She'd arranged a ride for a group of us in the high desert mountains above Santa Fe. Jim, the owner, announced that he had not fully tamed one of the horses. He asked for a volunteer. He had just enough horses to accommodate our group, and there were no substitutes. A man agreed to ride the horse, and right after he mounted him, the horse bolted and ran away. Jim galloped after them and led the horse back to our group with reins in hand. He then asked for another volunteer. Silence. More silence. I finally agreed to ride Feisty (my name for him). I know you're thinking this proves my judgment is questionable, and you may be right. As we proceeded forward, Feisty lurched, and I pulled back the reins. He reared up on his hind legs! Jim said calmly, "Oh, don't pull straight back. You have to give and take with this one." That was enlightening. I can't say I relaxed during the next 2 hours, though the panoramas were breathtaking. Perhaps the vistas were more beautiful because my moment-to-moment concentration was so intense, as I tested how much guidance this horse would receive from me. As I experimented with my body position, the angle I held the reins, and the pressure I applied with hand movements, we found a middle ground between us that made the ride possible.

From the time I was a kid, coming into union with a horse was bliss. I cried when I awoke from a dream that I'd been given a horse only to discover it wasn't real! I talked to my sister, Linda, about horse whisperers because she raises championship Arabian horses in pastures surrounded by the gorgeous Shenandoah Mountains in Virginia. She and her husband built their spacious barn with beautiful wood beams and light pouring in from slats in the ceiling. When a mare is pregnant, they watch her continually around the clock on closed circuit TV. When the time is right, they race to the barn to midwife the birth of an exquisite baby into the world. Linda studied with Clinton Anderson, one of the greatest horse whisperers, because she loves her magnificent

Arabians with the chiseled, aristocratic faces almost as much as her eight grandchildren.

Buck, a Film with Lessons for Psychotherapists

Buck would walk into a ring with a new horse he'd never met before, and the horse would exhibit aggressive and frightening behaviors to "create distance" from him (a common human defense). Buck explained that no one taught these horses how to be a member of their herd. You should walk sideways up to a horse as we use a graded approach when people become anxious or ashamed during human contact. We don't approach our anxious or defended clients directly and ask questions that can feel invasive without implicit and explicit permission, reading body signals, and adjusting our body language and vocal tones to create safety.

When Buck saw misbehavior (defenses) in a horse, he'd gently flap the horse's flank with some soft rags on a stick to slightly irritate the horse so he wouldn't like it but would also recognize that Buck meant no harm. My clients find it irritating when I interrupt to draw attention to self-protective habits that harm them, but such interventions are quite effective so long as the client has granted permission and participates as a collaborator. As with horses, our clients respond positively to clear messaging and kindness. Keeping our feedback consistent and timely is all-important until new behaviors and capacities form.

Many clinicians will understandably back away from creating irritations. Therapists want approval too. Yet, just like a "good enough horse whisperer" or a "good enough parent" or a "good enough therapist," we fail to help if we don't provide feedback that helps our clients find a better path. Some irritants are healing, and some are just plain annoying. What makes the difference?

Linda's recommendations:

- "It's ALL BODY LANGUAGE! Your eyes and face need to be soft. Your body needs to be RELAXED. (Relaxation requires self-care. We must allow for trial and error and the freedom to make mistakes, while giving caring attention to our shame and fear. When people push us away, it's usually due to their fear, shame, and suffering and not because of a deficiency within us.)

- Give instant praise when the horse (or human) is trying. Similarly, we can express appreciation for risky self-disclosure or attempts at a new behavior immediately.
- Horses (and humans) want to be safe and to please. Linda said, "You should have a happy tone to let a horse know you are delighted." She demonstrated with a lilting voice that was charming. As Buck said, "You love on 'em." Sense of mastery is a therapy outcome common factor. Highlighting the evidence of the client's growth encourages more change.
- Horses do not learn from pressure but rather from the "release from pressure," Linda said, "When you are trying to get a horse to move the forequarters, you tap gently on the neck with a stick. Usually, they will just move one front leg and you praise them with the stick by rubbing softly where you tapped them. Then tap again until they move and reward with a soft rub. Soon you will only have to carry the stick without tapping, and the horse will move. How fascinating! So, perhaps the positive reinforcement when a client drops a defense creates the learning experience? Something like, "You allowed me to feel close to you when you let me see your tears," provides the impetus to risk more emotional closeness.
- The trainer must perfectly time the release of pressure, or the horse becomes confused by the signals, which must be clear, decisive, and positive. Hope can plummet when the client doesn't recognize successes. If the therapist's response to change is slow, the client may feel lost and inadequate. The brain can more readily make links that lead to change when the therapist's input is timely and precise.
- Horses don't forget what they've learned! Neuroscience tells us that new attachment experiences alter brain structure over time, and our clients will not forget how to relate in the ways they've experienced with us!

The Power of Metaphor

People and horse whisperers rely upon language from the unconscious that arises from deep relaxation and receptivity to intuition. Perhaps metaphorical language falls between the cracks of verbal and non-verbal. Metaphors create images that penetrate the unconscious in ways that ordinary language does not. "Psychotherapists use many of the same devices as rhetoricians … vivid metaphors and sensory images that focus the patient's attention on ideas central to the therapeutic message. Successful therapists do this intuitively, but many could profit from more deliberate efforts to improve their communication with patients along these lines" (Frank & Frank, 1993).

Clients tell me that meaningful metaphors stick in their minds and inspire them into the future. Powerful metaphors in therapy evoke emotion and often spring from the creative collaboration of two unconscious minds. Interventions spoken without feeling, using abstract and predictable language, are less likely to be catalysts for change. As indicated by (Finlay, 2015), metaphorical language engages the whole self to make meaning in unforgettable ways:

> The value of engaging metaphors creatively and reflexively is emphasized, as various meanings of metaphors are often not self-evident. They need to be played with and worked through, both in dialogue and reverie. And they need to be seen in the broader context of individuals' histories, the therapeutic relationship, and the wider culture. The point that metaphors go beyond visual image to engage the different senses in multiple relational ways is highlighted. Although metaphors may be understood as being a function of language, in practice they arise through embodied intersubjective experiencing.
>
> (Finlay, 2015)

Metaphors are a universal language that is readily digestible and, therefore, less likely to evoke shame. Our clients can feel humiliated and "stupid" when we use jargon words that the client can't understand. Intellectualizing pulls the client further into a detached and distant state. Lyrical, vivid, or powerful imagery moves people from left-brain to right-brain, from the analytic mind into the feeling, intuitive, and receptive mind. I was delighted when a colleague exclaimed after viewing one of my sessions, "This work is chock full of metaphors!"

> As one gives oneself to being carried along by the affective cadence of the patient's session, one may sense its tone and subtleties. By being more open in this manner, to resonating to the patient, I find pictures forming in my creative zones; an image crystallizes, reflecting the patient's experience.
>
> (Hammer, 1990)

Some of my Favorite Metaphors

Children Knocking at the Door

The door to my consulting room is behind my client's chair. As I would face my client, I'd become aware of the door behind the person and envision children with small, muffled voices on the other side of the door. I could hear their tapping as they wished to gain entrance. I shared my fantasy with my clients that I sensed children inside them who were trying to gain our attention, requesting an invitation to enter and be seen. The imagery of children captured the innocence, pureness, and vulnerability of our feeling states that depend upon others' recognition to find healthy expression. Children also captured the tenderness I felt toward my client's feelings. My client and I were the big people, and the feeling children were small. I was on their side, and I would advocate for them. I hoped to persuade my client to do the same.

I might ask, "Do you hear them tapping on the other side of our door? Would you want to permit them to enter? They've been alone and unrecognized throughout your life. Do they deserve an audience with us, a real invitation to hang out with us, to be accepted as they are, and to be heard until they've had their say? When they are satisfied, they will leave. When they are not allowed entrance, do you think they will go quietly into the night? The answer is inevitably, "No. They will knock harder."

Parasitic Vines Wrapped around a Healthy Tree Trunk

When people express feeling overwhelmed by shame, anxiety, guilt, and negative self-protective strategies that drive their chronic anxiety, depression, or addictions, I love this metaphor of parasitic vines to represent these suffocating forces. I use this metaphor when people say, "That's just how I am." "I wouldn't know differently." "I've been this way all my life" These disabling internal forces are foreboding and dictatorial. I point out that my client is like the healthy tree trunk at their core that has become strangulated by parasitic vines (i.e., SAGSS). This metaphor often provides a startling revelation: "My symptoms of suffering are not me! My symptoms are like vines that have wrapped themselves around me through indoctrination and habit, but the part of me that observes these vines is separate from those forces." The "Parasitic vine" metaphor awakens the possibility to break free from the strangulating vines. When people absorb the meaning of the metaphor, many have said, "I feel hopeful for the first time in years."

Feelings are Forces of Nature

The metaphor, "Feelings are forces of nature," helps normalize emotions. Feelings accompany us at birth and are not of our choosing, serving a purpose if they are heeded. Like rainstorms or strong winds, feelings change and come to us as a gift. The nature metaphor has helped many clients to release guilt and shame over their feelings by normalizing them. I'll sometimes say, "I'm not talking to you, Barbara, but to your anger. Could we invite your anger into the room?" Barbara's anger may show up as a wild lioness, majestic and fierce. I once knew a hairstylist/ bouncer who encountered a thief in his garage. I gasped when he told me. He said to the intruder with glee, with his hands gesturing toward himself, "C'mon. Let me out of my cage!"

The River Wants to Flow

A man who I was sure would never cry shocked me by sobbing after I said, "The river wants to flow." He grew up on a riverbank, and I knew rivers were meaningful to him. Referencing specific phrases, memories, and details unique to an individual will land with more impact.

Our Emotional Rainbow

The shimmering rainbow is my metaphor for our awesome emotional repertoire. Feelings flow from one to the other with no real separation, as the colors of the rainbow merge into one spectacular vision. Why not embrace the awesome emotional rainbow that lives inside us and appreciate its power to make our lives meaningful and transcendent?

The Sherpa Therapist

I offer the metaphor "The Sherpa Therapist" to my trainees as a symbol for the equal and collaborative nature of our relationship to our clients.

The Sherpa doesn't make cold calls to convince someone of the joys of climbing and the superiority of one peak over another. The climber seeks out the Sherpa for expertise on the mountain of his choice, choosing someone who can be trusted with one's life. The Sherpa provides feedback about what we need to do to navigate the climb, offers warnings when we're in trouble, points out the best routes, and helps us gage our position and progress. What causes one climber to make it to the top and others to return to basecamp? That's a complex question. Climbers have different outcomes, but good Sherpas remain committed.

My Boa

As we discussed in Chapter 9, I had described a viciously critical and controlling part of a female client as a "boa constrictor." It was an invasive animal that choked and suffocated her. Most of the time, she'd engage in lush storytelling, but when she left this defense and started to move toward her feelings, she became short of breath and hyperfocused on her deficiencies. I helped her see these strangulating mechanisms as separate from her, and her new awareness created a dramatic shift in her. She began referencing her defensive processes as "My Boa," and she learned to pull this devouring creature off her.

A Magic Metaphor Day

I shall always treasure Metaphor Day in our training program, an event that was organized by our infinitely generous, imaginative, and innovative Training Program Coordinator, faculty member, and author of *Emotion Focused Workbook*, Bridget Quebodeaux, LMFT. She invited our trainees to bring a piece of art they'd created, signifying a metaphor they'd found to be potent in their work. Dr. Marks-Tarlow contributed a delightful piece to our Metaphor Art Exhibit (see Figure 11.1). She had read the following in an early draft from this book, "If a rainbow landed in your backyard, would you assign a value to one hue over another, critiquing and comparing each arc of this shimmering phenomenon? Or would you fall back in awe at this splendorous prism of light?"

Bridget brought in this next drawing of a panther, which she drew with the help of her son, Jackson, depicting a metaphor I'd used with

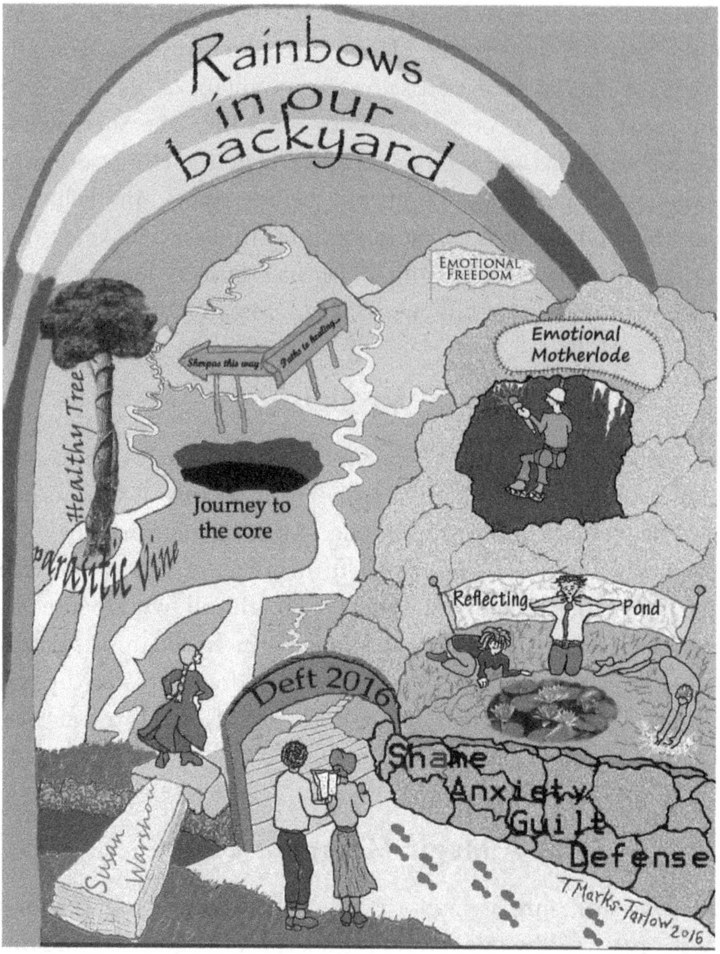

Figure 11.1
(Marks-Tarlow, 2016)

a suicidal client with memories of rape and desertion by both parents. As I sat with her profound sense of emptiness, despair, and deficiency, I told her I had a vision of a black panther stalking her psyche, casting a dark shadow of unworthiness over her life and her dreams. The panther was stealthy, sleek, and silent, and it prowled undetected. But now I could see it! Did she see it? This image resonated with her. She became aware of this force inside her for the first time, and we both observed how it bullied her. "Good!" I said. "Now

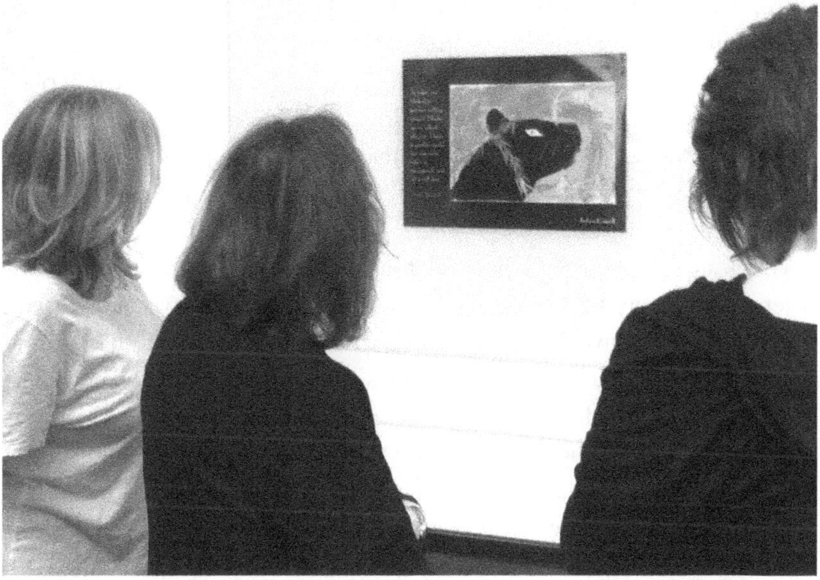

Figure 11.2 Black Panther

we can see it, so now we can track it! We have a freeze-frame!!" My client never forgot this image, and she used it to jar her awareness when she found herself at the mercy of her shame panther. Once she could recognize her panther in action, she began to gently push it back into the woods from whence it came.

This client made extraordinary progress overcoming her shame and began sharing her vulnerabilities and needs with those close to her. Revealing her dependencies was a huge accomplishment for her, such as telling a friend she'd felt forgotten when he didn't check on her after surgery. Such self-exposure was wholly new for her, and she was delighted she could communicate without casting-blame. Her depression ultimately disappeared.

People and Horses Sense Authenticity

Authenticity is consummately intuitive because it is spontaneous, natural and real. Therapists who are willing to be authentic must step outside of their defensive system and programmed responses. My sister's love for her horses is as real as it gets. She adopted a huge Premarin mare, a Percheron draft horse, headed for slaughter. When her mare arrived at 3:00 am, my sister greeted her in the pasture, lay next to her, and slept with her through the night. She named her horse "Lola," inspired by a line in a Barry Manilow song, "Whatever Lola wants, Lola gets." My sister nursed Lola to health. Lola was people-phobic but recognized true love when she felt it. Linda and Lola have a powerful attachment to this day.

People and horses regularly check for safety, and safety comes from consistency, a capacity to stay engaged, and authenticity. One woman with an intractable, vegetative depression came to me in desperation after several therapy attempts. She said, "Something is disarming about you, and I don't quite know what it is. But I haven't experienced this before and it gives me hope." Another client said, "I find you to be real. I've been to several therapists before and have had positive feelings and transferences, but this is different. You are like a real person. I haven't had this before, and that scares me." We began to notice her gaze aversion as she spoke. She then said that she'd never been so aware of how much shame and fear she had around being real in a relationship. A sample exchange:

Th: You know, I just noticed that I was about to tell you that I admire your courage to bravely tackle horrendous traffic and come here despite massive feelings of dread and hopelessness. But then I hesitated and considered not making this comment and wondered why? I anticipated you would push back. (*We both said the phrase "push back" at the same exact moment.*)

Ct: Yes! I agree that I would push back and invalidate your comment.

Th: I thought you would see me as dishonest and manipulative and find something wrong with me for thinking you had value.

Ct: (*Spoken with hesitation.*) I appreciate your comment. It shows me your vulnerability to risk exposing your real self to me.

This exchange brought forth tears as she realized the extent and the cost of her self-devaluation, which blocks others from appreciating her. These oppressive forces were in both of us, trying to steer us away from possible rejection. Compassion for herself arose as she became aware of the cost of her defenses. Both of us took a risk to share ourselves. She appreciated that I showed my caring for her by stepping outside my comfort zone.

We are all born to be authentic until human interaction chips away at this quality. We learn to become wily, strategic, and duplicitous, play roles, detach from ourselves, and become what we think people want us to be. The more we can reverse this learning, the more our relational gifts shine. My sister stressed the importance of relaxation while working with horses, and the same holds true for people. Therapists are more relaxed when we value our authentic selves. A graduate from the DEFT program told me that the most helpful parts were the ways "You helped me to be with myself."

Qualities of a People Whisperer

I encourage my trainees to:

- Accept what you don't know at present
- Appreciate what you do know
- Trust your intuition
- Take informed chances
- Share your observations
- Appreciate that you are like no other, as it should be
- Use the Healing Triad to support your well-being
- Express your creativity
- Recognize that failure is not a finality
- Stick with lifetime learning to build confidence
- Surround yourself with a supportive community

Risk and Failure

I lost a client today. Knowing that every partnership will not work allows me to relax while I work. I'm also willing to be an irritant in order to promote health, even when it brings challenges. The majority of wild and unruly horses responded to Buck as their trust grew, but some tortured animals could never be reached and remained violent. The horse I rode in Santa Fe could easily have traded me in at any moment, yet I'd committed to the ride and the risks it entailed. Choosing to take the next step and the one after that as we learn to become better therapists is all that is required. We will need compassion to forgive what we don't know. Showing care for ourselves embraces the vulnerability that allows us to connect. Self-compassion allows us see further into the complexities of the therapeutic relationship, as though we were wearing night goggles.

Self-compassion leads to other-compassion, and both inspired me to write this book. I had to find a way to write this book without an attachment to the outcome, allowing it to fail without seeing myself as a failure. Otherwise, I would not have written it for you. I still hope you will find it valuable, but I've also released any agendas. I'm now writing this book in earnest after entertaining the title, "The worst book ever written." I fantasized about having one chapter in the book filled with blank pages with the title, "Nothing Here" and the subtitle, "You thought I was kidding." Perfectionism was my enemy as an author, a teacher, and a therapist. Perhaps if I set out to do an awful job, or at least didn't care if I succeeded in failing, I'd at least take the next step. This freedom to experiment and fail is a prerequisite to becoming the best therapist we can be. Mark Manson addressed this well in *The Subtle Art of Not Giving a F*ck: A Counterintuitive Approach to Living a Good Life*. He said,

> The avoidance of suffering is a form of suffering. The avoidance of struggle is a struggle. Everything worthwhile in life is won through surmounting the associated negative experience. Any attempt to escape the negative, to avoid it or quash it or silence it, only backfires. The denial of failure is a failure. Hiding what is shameful is itself a form of shame.
>
> (Manson, 2016)

Pain is an inextricable thread in the fabric of life. When we attempt to get rid of that thread, we unravel everything else with it. In contrast, if we work with the pain, we become unstoppable. A dear client died recently and suddenly. My sobs told me how much I'd loved her. A colleague reflected that a therapist could attend a client's memorial service and feel as much grief as other attendees, yet we cannot talk about our profound relationship. We may be privy to dimensions of that person that few, if any, have seen. The therapists I've trained feel a sacred trust to serve their clients. They agonize when they fall short. You may be one of those people. When you care deeply to serve your clients well, and you take risks and persist in your efforts to use your best knowledge and intuition, and you do so with humility and deep feeling, nothing more is needed. Do not define yourself by your failures. May you feel joy and fulfillment in your contribution to the world.

References

Finlay, L. (2015). Sensing and making sense: Embodying metaphor in relational-centered psychotherapy. *The Humanistic Psychologist, 43*(4), 338–353. https://doi.org/10.1080/08873267.2014.993070

Frank, J. D., & Frank, J. B. (1993). *Persuasion and healing: A comparative study of psychotherapy*. Johns Hopkins University Press.

Hammer, E. (1990). *Reaching the affect: Style in the psychodynamic therapies*. Jason Aronson.

Manson, M. (2016). *The subtle art of not giving a f*ck: A counterintuitive approach to living a good life*. Harper.

Marks-Tarlow, T. (2012). *Norton series on interpersonal neurobiology. Clinical intuition in psychotherapy: The neurobiology of embodied response*. W. W Norton & Co.

EPILOGUE

Dynamic Emotion Focused Therapy (DEFT)

Dynamic Emotion Focused Therapy (DEFT), developed by Susan Warren Warshow, emerged from two decades of clinical observation, client feedback, and study of the literature regarding the effects of dysregulated shame reactions on the therapeutic alliance and outcome. DEFT interventions place *shame sensitivity* at the forefront, especially when dealing with the barriers to core feelings and emotional intimacy, i.e., toxic forms of shame, anxiety, guilt, and self-protective strategies (SAGSS). The Healing Triad is employed to move beyond these obstacles (see Chapter 5). The approach seeks to transfer the therapist's compassion for the client's relational trauma through embodied and verbal responses that allow the client to internalize self-compassion (the Therapeutic Transfer of Compassion for Self or TTCS).

Key Features of Dynamic Emotion Focused Therapy

- The therapist practices *shame sensitivity* in all interactions through the following:
  - A Replacing shame with compassion. All defensive responses are survival-based, and the therapist's implicit and explicit responses need to reflect the tragic cost of the client's defenses.
  - B Giving attention to the impact of prosody, body language, facial expression, and eye gaze. There are times when all therapists

must work to achieve genuine compassion for the client, which is essential in transmitting acceptance, safety, and empathy.

C Briefly self-disclosing and sharing vulnerability for the purpose of reducing the client's sense of aloneness and increasing the connection between both partners.

D Relinquishing the role of expert, e.g., collaboratively seeking a focus and making meaning of the therapeutic experience.

E Highlighting the developmental context of defenses, i.e., protective and resourceful mechanisms/habits unconsciously incorporated in childhood. The approach does not "turn against" the defenses but instead suggests releasing "self-protective" strategies that inflict harm.

F Framing defenses as neither intentional nor fixed parts of oneself, but rather as learned, automatic mechanisms that can be left behind.

G Avoiding shaming language, e.g., "You're digressing again," or "Why would you want to do that?" or "You're building a wall," which suggests blame.

H Instilling hope by emphasizing strengths when drawing attention to defenses. E.g., "You've successfully broken other habits in your life."

I Supporting the therapist's willingness to self-reflect without self-devaluation, be vulnerable, and participate in the growth process, crucial factors in a *shame sensitive* therapeutic relationship. All humans suffer from trauma and deserve compassion, including therapists.

- Invites the client to clarify specific goals for therapy throughout the process; offers a path to overcoming defenses against visualizing dreams and desires; and urges rapid identification and response to waning hope in the therapy process.
- Clarifies and seeks agreement on the client's role and the therapist's role in the therapeutic alliance. An egalitarian, collaborative, respectful, and non-authoritative partnership strengthens an individuated sense of self.
- Employs the Healing Triad in partnership with the client to transcend toxic SAGSS (**awareness** of SAGSS), **transfer of compassion**, and **will.** The latter represents the intention to direct caring attention

toward one's internal experience, embrace feelings, and connect with self and others.

- Tracks and attends to the physiological sensations and language of toxic shame, anxiety, and guilt. Shame often has similar manifestations to anxiety and needs to be recognized and titrated in similar ways.
- Distinguishes the self-limiting from self-enhancing parts of the self with the client's help when encountering SAGSS.
- Sustains a focus on feelings with the client's permission and processes complex unconscious emotions. DEFT views ALL feelings as valuable, neither positive nor negative, but rather having a purpose.
- Consolidates the insights resulting from emotion processing and explores the practical application of the therapeutic experience.

DEFT Principles of Practice

- Embraces attachment theory. All interventions seek to convey compassion, safety, and respect through verbal and non-verbal embodied responses.
- Highlights the client's strengths over deficits.
- Recognizes challenging types of self-disclosure and emotional engagement as "breakthroughs to intimacy" worthy of celebration.
- Regards full breakthroughs to complex feelings are only one of many powerful elements in healing.
- Recommends that therapists place intense emotional breakthroughs in perspective as one path to healing and to appreciate every instance of increased emotional engagement and interaction that the client finds valuable.
- Distinguishes between feeling compassion and expressing compassion in a way that the client can internalize.
- Draws clear distinctions between the therapist's and the client's roles, reminding therapists that they are one-half of the therapeutic partnership and must not take full responsibility for the outcome.
- Reinforces therapist spontaneity, creativity, and authenticity – stepping outside of any model or protocol – to bring one's unique self to the therapeutic relationship.

- Engages in play and humor, which can help reduce defense and form connection.
- Uses vivid language and metaphor to enhance the impact of therapeutic concepts (e.g., we might describe the SAGSS system to a client as a "parasitical vine wrapped around an otherwise healthy tree trunk").
- Highly values clinical intuition and "instinctive knowing," alongside theoretical grounding.
- Offers an explicit invitation to explore cultural differences between the therapist and client and their impact on the therapeutic relationship.
- Welcomes and explores spiritual or religious experiences initiated by the client and related to the client's emotional health.
- Views the origins of trauma as stemming not only from the family of origin but also from cultural, religious, peer group, educational, and other experiences (e.g., racial discrimination, socio-economic shaming, severe childhood bullying, gang cultures, abusive institutions, poverty, the horrors of war, irresolvable medical conditions, and physical disabilities). We advise therapists to carefully explore the history of the individual's suffering without preconceptions.
- DEFT resists strict adherence to any model, including its own. The complex mystery of the human psyche is never to be fully known; therefore, DEFT embraces a state of humility in the therapist, believing the response to intervention provides the information that matters the most.

INDEX

Page numbers in *italics* refer to figures.